Creative

Clinical

Teaching

in the

Health

Professions

Creative
Clinical
Teaching

in the

Health
Professions

Sherri Melrose,

Caroline Park,

AND *Beth Perry*

◊ AU PRESS

Published by AU Press, Athabasca University
1200, 10011 – 109 Street
Edmonton, AB
T5J 3S8

https://doi.org/10.15215/aupress/9781771993319.01

Cover design by Sergiy Kozakov
Printed and bound in Canada

Library and Archives Canada Cataloguing in Publication
Title: Creative clinical teaching in the health professions / Sherri Melrose, Caroline
Park, and Beth Perry.
Names: Melrose, Sherri, 1951– author. | Park, Caroline, 1948– author. | Perry, Beth,
1957– author.
Description: Includes bibliographical references.
Identifiers: Canadiana (print) 20210228032 | Canadiana (ebook) 20210228156 | ISBN
9781771993319 (softcover) | ISBN 9781771993326 (PDF) | ISBN 9781771993333 (EPUB)
Subjects: LCSH: Medicine—Study and teaching. | LCSH: Medical personnel—
In-service training.
Classification: LCC R834 .M45 2021 | DDC 610.71/1—DC23

We acknowledge the financial support of the Government of Canada through the
Canada Book Fund (CBF) for our publishing activities and the assistance provided
by the Government of Alberta through the Alberta Media Fund.

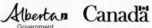

To our students, who teach us to be better teachers and better people.
To our colleagues, who inspire us with their dedication to teaching excellence.
To our university, for giving us the freedom to be innovators.
To our families, for providing us with encouragement and purpose.

Contents

Acknowledgements

We are grateful to Pamela Holway, Connor Houlihan, Karyn Wisselink, and Megan Hall at Athabasca University Press for their guidance and support.

We extend our sincere thanks to the following clinical teachers who graciously shared their wisdom through the practical "From the Field" suggestions offered throughout the book: Mary Ellen Bond, Lynda Champoux, Amelia Chauvette, Teresa Evans, Mary Ann Fegan, Jacqueline Mann, Mary Ann Morris, Cathy Schoales, Kara Sealock, and Adrienne Weare.

Creative

Clinical

Teaching

in the

Health

Professions

Theoretical Foundations of Teaching and Learning

I am not a teacher; only a fellow traveler of whom you asked the way.
I pointed ahead—ahead of myself as well as of you.
GEORGE BERNARD SHAW (N.D., N.P.)

Some educators might share George Bernard Shaw's (1908) notion that teaching is about learning with students as fellow travellers. Others might see the process of teaching in entirely different ways. However, few educators would disagree with Shaw's view that the practice of teaching involves pointing ahead through intentional processes that facilitate learning. Clinical teachers can guide learners with the help of established theoretical foundations from the discipline of education.

Theoretical foundations in the discipline of education include understanding and valuing how to integrate scholarship into the practice of teaching. They also include knowing how to apply conceptual frameworks, theories, and models. *Conceptual frameworks* are overarching views of the world. They differ from theories in that they are often more abstract and enduring than theories. *Theories* tend to offer more immediate, practical, and factual guidance. They are more adaptable to change and might or might not be useful, depending on the circumstances. *Models* offer even more specific direction and are often represented visually in a diagram or chart.

Theoretical foundations include terms such as "educate," "pedagogy," and "andragogy." The word *educate* comes from the Latin *educere*, which means to draw out and develop (Educate, n.d.). *Pedagogy*, the art and science of education, seeks to understand practices and methods of instruction that can help teachers to educate or draw out learners (About Education, n.d.). Although pedagogy seeks to understand how to teach learners of all ages, *andragogy* is the study of helping adults to learn (Knowles, 1984). Students enrolled in health-care programs in postsecondary or higher education institutions are considered adult learners.

Historically, higher education in general (and clinical teaching in particular) placed little importance on the actual practice of how to teach. Professors and instructors in postsecondary institutions were honoured more for knowledge of subject matter within their discipline than for instructional methods. However, since the time of Socrates, scholars of education have examined how learning occurs, which instructional practices facilitate learning, and the contexts in which learning occurs best. Today content knowledge alone is not enough—clinical teachers must ground their practice in an understanding of educational processes. In this chapter, we provide a brief introduction to the scholarship of teaching and learning, common conceptual frameworks, and adult education theories and models. In each section, we include creative practical strategies that educators in the health professions can readily use in their everyday clinical teaching practice.

THE SCHOLARSHIP OF TEACHING AND LEARNING

In 1990, Ernest Boyer, then the president of the Carnegie Foundation for Teaching, challenged an existing norm in higher education. Traditionally, university educators—known as the "professoriate" or the "academy"—were expected to demonstrate their scholarship primarily by researching and publishing in their areas of content expertise. In his seminal publication, *Scholarship Reconsidered: Priorities of the Professoriate*, Boyer called for a broader definition of scholarship that recognizes excellent teaching and content area research as equally important. He proposed four separate yet overlapping functions of scholarship: the scholarship of discovery, the scholarship of integration, the scholarship of application, and the scholarship of teaching. Boyer defined the different forms of scholarship as follows.

The scholarship of discovery comes closest to what is meant when academics speak of "research.". . . No tenets in the academy are held in higher regard than the commitment to knowledge for its own sake. . . . [It is] central to the work of higher learning . . . and contributes not only to the stock of human knowledge but also to the intellectual climate of college or university.

The scholarship of integration underscores the need for scholars who give meaning to isolated facts, . . . making connections across disciplines, placing the specialties in larger context, illuminating data in a revealing way . . . [It is] serious, disciplined work that seeks to interpret, draw together, and bring new insight to bear on original research. . . . [It] fit[s] one's research—or the research of others—into larger intellectual patterns.

The scholarship of application moves toward engagement . . . [and] reflect[s] the Zeitgeist of the nineteenth and early twentieth century that . . . land grant colleges . . . were founded on the principle that higher education must serve the interests of the larger community. . . . [It is] tied to one's special field of knowledge and relate[s] to, and flow[s] directly out of, this professional activity, . . . requiring the vigor—and the accountability—traditionally associated with research activities.

Finally, we come to *the scholarship of teaching*. . . . As a scholarly enterprise, teaching begins with what the teacher knows. . . . Those who teach must, above all, be well informed, and steeped in the knowledge of their fields. . . . Teaching is also a dynamic endeavor involving all analogies, metaphors, and images that build bridges between the teacher's understanding and the student's learning. . . . Yet, today teaching is often viewed as a routine function, tacked on, something almost anyone can do. . . . Defined as scholarship, however, teaching both educates and entices future scholars . . . and keeps the flame of scholarship alive (p.14–25).

The evolving definition of scholarship later came to include six expectations. To be considered scholarly, teachers' work must demonstrate clear goals, adequate preparation, appropriate methods, significant results, effective presentation, and reflective critique (Glassick, 2000; Glassick et al., 1997).

As the scholarship of teaching became more widely known, Lee Shulman (1998), another president of the Carnegie Foundation, extended the definition further by introducing four important standards. Work must be (1) made public in some manner; (2) have been subjected to peer review by members of one's intellectual or professional community; (3) citable, refutable, and able to be built upon; and (4) shared among members of that community.

As the importance of roles for learners in the process of teaching also gained recognition, Boyer's (1990) scholarship of teaching continued to evolve and is now referred to as the scholarship of teaching and learning. Journals such as the *International Journal for the Scholarship of Teaching and Learning*, *Journal of the Scholarship of Teaching and Learning*, *Canadian Journal for the Scholarship of Teaching and Learning*, and Canadian Association of Schools of Nursing (CASN) *Quality Advancement in Nursing Education* are examples of refereed journals committed to public dissemination of teachers' scholarly work. Educators in nursing (Cash & Tate, 2012; Duncan et al., 2014; Oermann, 2015), pharmacy (Gubbins, 2014), physical therapy (Anderson & Tunney, 2014), and other health professions are making concerted efforts to apply the scholarship of teaching and learning to both clinical and academic areas of practice.

In Canada, CASN (2013) developed a seminal position statement on scholarship. This statement adapts Boyer's (1990) model of scholarship and includes the scholarship of teaching as an activity expected of nurse educators.

A Strategy to Try ▶ *Everyday Scholarship*
Imagine a new way to solve a common teaching dilemma or to introduce an innovation into your clinical teaching practice. Consider the standards of scholarship as you think through the issues involved. How can you make public the solutions that you develop or the innovations that you create so others can benefit? How can you invite peers to review them? How and where can you cite the explanations of what you have done so others can know about them, refute them, or extend them?

Invitational Theory

William Purkey (1992) put forward invitational theory as an educational framework of learning and teaching relationships based on human value, responsibility, and capability. Invitational learning is observed in the social context, in which learners should be invited by the teacher to develop their potentials. The four pillars of invitational theory are respect, trust, optimism, and intentionality. The invitational instructor invites learners in, welcomes them, creates warm and welcoming educational environments, provides optimum learning opportunities, and bids them a warm farewell at the conclusion of the learning experience.

In 1983, Parker Palmer introduced the term "invitational classroom." He emphasized that "an air of hospitality" facilitates the inviting environment (1983/1993, p. 71). Hospitality in his words means "receiving each other, our struggles, our newborn ideas, with openness and care" (p. 74). Palmer concluded that both teachers and learners experience positive consequences when the classroom is invitational (see 1983/1993, 1998, 2007).

A Strategy to Try ▶ *Meaningful Introductions*

To be true to invitational theory, the instructor needs to find ways to welcome learners to the course as a great host would welcome guests to a dinner party. Introductions are important if you adopt the invitational theory viewpoint.

Rather than having learners just say their names, consider inviting them to share a special object (e.g., their favourite teacup or a picture of their special place). This will create fodder for discussion, help each person to feel like an individual, and promote connections among learners in the group.

Constructivism

Constructivist thinking, as espoused by seminal educationalists such as Jean Piaget (1972) and Lev Vygotsky (1978), suggests that knowledge is constructed by learners themselves. Those who view the world through a constructivist lens believe that learners bring valuable existing knowledge to their learning experiences. They view the role of the teacher as building on that knowledge by providing personally meaningful activities.

Constructivist teachers also believe that learning will be enhanced by interactions with informed others such as teachers, practitioners, and peers. Therefore, an important aspect of any constructivist teacher's practice is to plan for and facilitate opportunities for helpful social interaction. In clinical teaching environments, instructors who use a constructivist conceptual perspective will create impactful connections individually with students and ensure that opportunities for connections with other students and staff members are possible.

Melrose et al. (2013, p. 71) summarize constructivism as a conceptual framework:

> Constructivist learning environments incorporate consensually validated knowledge and professional practice standards, and competencies are comprehensively evaluated. Students' misconceptions are identified and redirected. Learners are viewed as having a unique and individual zone of ability where they are able to complete an activity independently. Working collaboratively, students and teachers determine what assistance is needed to move toward increasing that zone of independence.

Instructional scaffolding. Just as carpenters use scaffolds to support and prop up buildings during the construction process, so too educators use scaffolds to support learners temporarily. Scaffolds might be needed the most at the beginnings of learning experiences and are gradually decreased as students become increasingly able to achieve learning outcomes independently (Hagler et al., 2011; Morgan & Brooks, 2012; Sanders & Welk, 2005).

Scaffolds initially provide substantive foundational knowledge, offer sequenced opportunities for understanding new ideas, and are gradually withdrawn as learners construct their own ways of understanding the material. Learning activities are designed to link to students' personal goals, connect theory to practice, and invite deep and critical reflection.

Clinical teachers can expect that instructional scaffolds such as a syllabus, course outcomes, and required evaluation activities are in place for student groups. However, each clinical area offers unlimited possibilities for additional innovative scaffolds. For example, clinical teachers can create specific activities for their clinical agency placement areas. They can tailor orientation activities to fit their specific practicum placement areas. They can create advance organizers such as concept maps and mind maps (Melrose et al., 2013) illustrating approaches to patient care or procedures that students will implement. Clinical teachers can also sketch simple diagrams to supplement verbal or textual instructions. They can pose thought-provoking questions that invite learners to view the world in new ways (Nevers & Melrose, 2016). They can model procedures and invite students to participate as much as they are able, turning the activity over to students themselves whenever possible. Clinical teachers can share their own clinical experiences, both those that involved clear professional responses and those that were ambiguous and without clear answers. Woodley (2015) suggests creating individualized orientation folders, either paper or electronic, to distribute to students at the beginning of their clinical rotation.

A Strategy to Try ▶ *Craft a Catchy Mnemonic*
Mnemonics are memory aids that use the first letters of a set of words to form sequences of information that are easy to remember. One example is the well-known A B C of resuscitation, A for airway, B for breathing, and C for circulation. You can craft a catchy mnemonic to help learners in your area remember critical points. Select three to five important pieces of information about a common condition or procedure. Choose one word to represent each of these critical points. Include at least one word starting with a vowel if possible. Share your mnemonic with students early in the clinical experience and encourage all members of the group to refer to it during discussions.

Before each clinical practicum, arrange a private one-to-one meeting with each of your students. Draw from the following "getting to know you" set of questions to guide your discussions.

- What is your style of learning?
- What are some of your strengths and challenges?
- What are your expectations of your instructor?
- How can I help you as a learner?
- How will I know when you are anxious, stressed, or nervous?
- What are you looking forward to in this upcoming practice experience?
- Why did you go into your professional field, and where do you see yourself after completing your program?
- Do you have any health professionals in your family or any experience in your field yourself?
- Do you work outside of school?
- What are your hobbies or interests?
- Any other concerns I can address at this point?

LYNDA CHAMPOUX, BSN, INSTRUCTOR, AND COLLEAGUES,
DEPARTMENT OF NURSING, CAMOSUN COLLEGE

Transformational Learning

Adult educator Jack Mezirow (1978, 1981, 1997, 2009) is credited with articulating transformational learning as a framework for teaching and learning. This worldview suggests that learning involves meaningful and transformative shifts in students' established beliefs and assumptions. These shifts are expected to occur when disorienting dilemmas arise. In other words, learners can experience profound transformations when they have been deeply affected by a learning experience. Clinical learning environments offer limitless opportunities for both teachers and students to think in new and different ways and to experience transformational learning.

Teachers who ground their practice in transformative learning find ways to challenge learners. They look for clinical experiences that can trigger new insights and invite critical reflection. These teachers encourage students to question what they believe to be true. They also expect students to question what they are taught and what they see in practice. Critical thinking and critical reflection are key elements of this conceptual framework.

Critical thinking. Critical thinking involves analyzing, assessing, and reconstructing (Critical Thinking Community, n.d.). Individuals who think critically seek relevant information and make judgments, interpretations, and inferences based on evidence and context (Brookfield, 2012; Burrell, 2014; Hansson, 2019; Rowles, 2012; Turner, 2005; Zygmont & Moore Schaefer, 2006). Socrates was one of the first educators to espouse the use of questioning methods by teachers (Socratic questioning) to require learners to think deeply, challenge their own assumptions, and gather evidence before accepting new ideas (Paul & Elder, 2007). Two clinical teaching activities that promote critical thinking are reflective journalling and case studies.

Critical reflection. Clinical components or programs in health professions often use *reflective journalling*. As an assignment, it is well suited to adult learners, helps to bridge the theory-to-practice gap, and can promote reflective practice (Chelliah & Zain, 2016; Garrity, 2013). The process fosters development of higher order thinking skills (Jarvis & Baloyi, 2020) and promotes personal and professional growth, empowerment, and development of knowledge, skills, and attitudes (Garrity, 2013). As a transformative learning approach, reflective journalling creates needed introspective opportunities for students to identify and analyze their feelings of discomfort, stress, or anxiety (Ganzer & Zauderer, 2013; Waldo & Hermanns, 2009).

Journals are often used as a tool for student evaluation (Ekelin et al., 2021; Lasater & Nielsen, 2009; Ross et al., 2014; Waldo & Hermanns, 2009). Including reflective journalling in evaluation is a key advantage for students, providing an opportunity for them to articulate and share the experiences that transformed or shifted their thinking. Teachers or clinical staff members might not otherwise be aware of these experiences or their profound impacts. With reflective journalling, students can think critically, be creative, express personal views, and critique their own performance.

Yet an expected disadvantage of evaluating reflective journalling is the reluctance of students to self-critique fully and honestly if doing so might affect the grades that they receive. Teachers can find it difficult to mark journals objectively, and reviewing them can be time consuming (Chan, 2009). Guidelines for implementing reflective journalling assignments include providing clear explanations of what critical reflection means, what the approximate length of journal entries should be, how often they should be submitted, and the extent of privacy and confidentiality that students can expect (Chan, 2009). Timely feedback on student journal entries strengthens the reflective process.

A Strategy to Try ▶ *Critical Reflection: What It Is and What It Is Not*
Differentiating between reflective journal entries demonstrating critical thinking and those simply recording activities and observations might not be easy for students. If reflective journalling is used in your program, or you wish to invite students to journal, show them what critical reflection is. Provide examples of journal entries that demonstrate introspection, self-critique, and experiences of feeling distressed or anxious. Emphasize the importance of reflecting honestly on what went well and what could or should be done differently next time. To illustrate what critical reflection is not, also provide examples of entries that are more superficial and do not really indicate shifts in thinking or a willingness to look at issues in new ways.

Case studies or case methods are also widely used during clinical components of programs for health professions. Case studies promote critical thinking, problem solving, self-direction, active learning, and communication skills (Carnegie Mellon, n.d.; Gaberson et al., 2015; Popil, 2011; Tomey, 2003).

Case studies are stories of real-life situations with complexities, dilemmas, and issues that are more abstract than concrete. Details in case studies are important, and the information presented must be specific. "Correct" responses and professional actions should not immediately be apparent. This lack of clarity provides learners with opportunities to practise identifying the kinds of problems that are present, to suggest different treatment approaches, and, most importantly, to consider new points of view (Carnegie Mellon, n.d.).

Clinical teachers can draw from their own experiences to create case studies, or they can access fully developed and peer-reviewed cases posted on health-care resources websites. When judging the merit of a case study for use in a specific area, assess whether the client situation and the setting are realistic and whether the information provided is detailed but brief. Discussion questions accompanying the cases should be open ended, inviting critiques and inspiring questions about the additional information that learners need to seek (Carnegie Mellon, n.d). Supplementing any case study activity with background information, such as anatomical and physiological reviews, lab test information, or excerpts from required texts, will help students to solve problems posed within the case in more informed ways.

A Strategy to Try ▶ *Draft a Case Study*
Reflect on your own experiences as you first began working in the area where you now teach. Does a particular case stand out? Why? As a new practitioner, what was difficult or perplexing about this case? How did you and other members of the health-care team try to resolve dilemmas associated with the case? What did you try that worked? What did not work? What did you wish you had known then that you know now? How did you go about finding the additional information you needed?

Write out the key details as briefly as possible as a draft case study. Separately, write out discussion questions and supplemental theoretical information. Ask your colleagues to review your draft case study, share it with different groups of students, and revise it as necessary. When your draft case study is consistently well received, consider submitting it for publication on an open educational resource website such as MERLOT (MERLOT Health Sciences, n.d.). By publicly sharing your well-received case study, you will strengthen your own scholarship and provide other clinical teachers with a useful teaching tool.

Indigenous Ways of Knowing

It is beyond the scope of this book to provide an in-depth exploration of the many experiences that contribute to Indigenous ways of knowing. Considerable diversity exists among Indigenous peoples around the world, and our aim is simply to offer a sampling of some of the assumptions and beliefs that might undergird some Indigenous worldviews. As a way of inviting educators in the health professions to explore ideas associated with Indigenous thinking further (and in their own ways), we introduce the concepts of "coming to know" and "holistic thinking" with brief comments on each.

Coming to know is a key concept within many Indigenous worldviews. It emphasizes a process of reflecting deeply and personally and of finding a balance between Indigenous knowing and Western perspectives (Snively & Williams, 2016). This reflective process requires people to undertake both formal and informal learning tasks by calming their minds, turning their thoughts inward, and establishing a mindset that seeks to reveal a sense of harmony with nature. The experience of coming toward (or coming to) learning includes a belief that people have gained valuable wisdom from their ancestors and that it will support them in approaching tasks with an open mind and a kind heart and spirit (Snively & Williams, 2016).

Holistic thinking also plays an important role in Indigenous ways of knowing. Holistic (or wholistic) perspectives view people as whole beings, with interconnections among all aspects of their physical, emotional, spiritual, and intellectual selves (Cull et al., 2018). These interconnections extend beyond individuals and emphasize respect for, and connections to, the land. High value is also placed on belonging and on relationships with others, including family members, communities, and nations (Cull et al., 2018). Teaching approaches that include storytelling (discussed further in Chapter 5), and opportunities for Elders to share oral traditions, support holistic thinking.

Holistic thinking is reflected in a set of learning principles articulated by the First Nations Education Steering Committee (n.d.), the group collaborated with Indigenous elders, scholars, and knowledge keepers to develop the following nine principles that reflect Indigenous ways of learning:

1. Learning ultimately supports the well-being of the self, the family, the community, the land, the spirits, and the ancestors.
2. Learning is holistic, reflexive, reflective, experiential, and relational (focused on connectedness, on reciprocal relationships, and on a sense of place).
3. Learning involves recognizing the consequences of one's actions.
4. Learning involves generational roles and responsibilities.
5. Learning recognizes the role of Indigenous knowledge.
6. Learning is embedded in memory, history, and story.
7. Learning involves patience and time.
8. Learning requires exploration of one's identity.
9. Learning involves recognizing that some knowledge is sacred and only shared with permission and or in certain situations.

The developers of these principles acknowledged that, though the principles do not capture the realities and experiences of all Indigenous peoples, they do reflect the common values about and perspectives on education held by one Canadian group (Alberta Regional Professional Development Consortium, 2018; First Nations Education Steering Committee, n.d.). Educators can apply the principles as a foundation for increasing their understanding of some of the commonalities and cultural constructs inherent in Indigenous ways of knowing.

A Strategy to Try ▶ *Learn More about Indigenous Ways of Knowing*
Which resources are available in your educational institution, clinical setting, or community that could help you to learn more about Indigenous ways of knowing? Which support services or organizations are available to Indigenous students or health professionals? Initiate contact with one of these organizations and explore ways to create collaborations. For example, develop a list of guest speakers who would be willing to join your clinical group during a post-conference (virtually or in person). Or subscribe to a newsletter and note any public activities of interest to you or your students.

Since Malcolm Knowles (1980, p. 43) labelled andragogy as the "art and science of helping adults learn," theorists in adult education continue to contribute important ideas about how teachers can best facilitate learning among adults. Many of these ideas or emerging theories are well suited to clinical learning environments, in which practitioners in their workplaces are actively working with both clients and students.

Assumptions underlying andragogy as an educational approach (Knowles 1975, 1980, 1984) are that adult learners are independent and self-directed. They bring accumulated life experiences that are rich resources for learning. Adults' learning needs are closely related to their changing social roles. Adults are motivated by internal rather than external factors. They are problem centred and most interested in immediate application of knowledge. For younger learners and those with little existing knowledge of a topic, some teaching might need to be more teacher-directed than self-directed. However, most adult educational experiences are grounded in a climate of acceptance, respect, and support, with learners expected to be actively involved in co-creating their learning. In the following paragraphs, we discuss three foundational elements of andragogy: self-direction, experiential learning, and collaboration.

Self-Direction

Self-direction is a foundational element of andragogy. Individuals who are self-directed accept responsibility for their learning by selecting, managing, and assessing many of the activities that they need throughout their learning process (Brookfield, 1984; Guglielmino, 2014; International Society for Self-Directed Learning, n.d.; Knowles, 1975). Many practicum students in the health professions had their previous learning experiences directed by teachers who told them what to do, what to study, and which goals to achieve. When students have had limited opportunities to assume responsibility for their own learning, clinical instructors can help by clearly communicating that self-direction is expected and required. For example, instructors can ask "How do you direct your own learning and how can we best help in that effort?" (Douglass & Morris, 2014, p. 13).

Think about a time when you needed to implement a new clinical activity, but instructions weren't available. What did you do? How did you select resources or information to guide you? What did you do with these resources to manage them or piece them together? How did you assess your process and determine that you could go ahead and safely implement the activity?

Self-direction involves selecting, managing, and assessing what's needed to be able to say "I can do that." In a group discussion, explain your own process of self-direction to students. Using the questions above, invite students to share examples of how they went about learning a new task. Close the activity by emphasizing the importance of self-direction in clinical learning environments.

Experiential Learning

Experiential learning, also termed "hands on" or "learning by doing," is a second foundational element of andragogy. Experiential learning theory suggests that, when learners are directly immersed in activities and then reflect analytically on their experiences, the process can integrate cognitive, emotional, and physical functions (Association for Experiential Education, n.d.; Dewey, 1938; Kolb, 1984). Each learner's experience is uniquely personal and will vary with context.

Teachers can support experiential learning by becoming involved in learners' ways of analyzing their experiences. Teachers can guide learners toward thinking beyond just the local contexts of their experiences (Moon, 2004). For example, Jacobson and Ruddy (2004) suggest posing questions such as Did you notice. . . ? Why did that happen? Does that happen in life? Why does that happen? How can you use that?

David Kolb (1984; Kolb & Fry, 1975) created an enduring model to explain experiential learning. He theorized that learning is a spiralling process of four steps. First, learners carry out an action or have a concrete experience. Second, they think about or reflect on that action in relation to that specific situation. Third, they try to understand the abstract concepts involved and look for ways to generalize beyond the specific situation. Fourth, they apply the knowledge and test what they discovered in new situations.

Practitioners in different clinical areas do not all do things in the same way. When students are implementing clinical activities in one placement area, they can find it challenging to generalize accurately beyond that specific situation. To encourage students to think broadly about what they are learning from what they are doing and how that knowledge might be applied to other situations, suggest that they develop a keeper file.

A keeper file is a collection of notes that students believe will be valuable in their future practice. Each note in the file includes a brief reflection on a clinical activity that they implemented in their present practicum. It should also include relevant theoretical thinking. Most importantly, though, it should include why students thought that being able to do this activity was a keeper. What did they learn in this practicum that can be generalized and applied in other clinical experiences and in their future practice?

Collaboration

A third foundational element of andragogy is replacing the hierarchy between teachers and students with collaboration and shared responsibility (Brookfield, 1986; Brookfield & Preskill, 2005; Imel, 1991). Traditional university programs presented information primarily through didactic methods such as lectures and assigned readings. Motivation was extrinsic, usually in the form of grades. Students often worked alone and might have felt that they were in competition with their peers. However, as ideas from the field of adult education are integrated into higher education settings, shifts are occurring. Students are now more familiar with the notion that they are expected to be active participants in their learning. Motivation is becoming more intrinsic, and most university students have experience working in small groups (Kurczek & Johnson, 2014). Integrating collaboration among students and having them work together in clinical practice areas can be an effective instructional approach and one that is relatively easy to apply. In contrast, establishing a learning environment in which the hierarchy between teachers and students is eliminated is less straightforward. Ultimately, teachers evaluate students. Still, teachers' relationships with students in higher education programs can be collaborative.

In academic settings, the teaching role is changing from authoritative professor to learning facilitator. One example is King's (1993, p. 30) seminal call for teachers in higher education to be more like a "guide on the side" than a "sage on the stage." Daloz (2012) urges higher education teachers to create mentoring relationships with students. Competitive thinking among students can be reduced by pass or fail grading systems rather than numeric or letter grades (Kohn, 2012; Melrose, 2017; White, 2010). In clinical settings, teachers are investing more in their relationships with students and making efforts to facilitate discussions rather than simply transmit knowledge (Beckman & Lee, 2009). Collaborative learning is not a matter of expert teachers transmitting knowledge to amateurs; rather, it is teachers and students working together to pursue knowledge (Barkley et al., 2005; Palmer, 2007).

Clinical teachers can collaborate and share responsibility for learning by inviting students to take on leadership roles within their clinical groups. In the following two "From the Field" strategies, instructors provide direction for activities that can help to facilitate collaboration.

From the Field   *Take a Turn at Team Leading*

Most teams of health professionals working together in institutions or agencies have someone designated as the team leader. This is often a rotating position. That is, someone is assigned to the role for a certain period, and then another person takes on the role. Often the team leader is someone who has several years of experience.

During their clinical placement experience, students can practise being the team leader for other students in their clinical group. Usually, a clinical group of approximately eight students will work a shift on the same unit. This is how the activity is organized.

- Each week during the clinical placement a student is assigned the role of team leader.
- The student who is acting as team leader arrives 15 minutes early for the shift to review the patients whom each student in the group will be caring for on that shift. The student team leader talks to the nurse in charge and makes certain that the patients whom the students are caring for are stable and appropriate to be assigned to student nurses.

- During the shift, the student team leader uses leadership skills to remind the other students on the team about matters such as changes in doctors' orders, incoming laboratory results, documentation requirements, discharge planning, and maintenance of professional standards. The student team leader organizes breaks and ensures that coverage is appropriate. The leader also provides feedback to and support for team members and acts as the liaison between the instructor and each student on the team.

Note that, if the student group is too large for one student team leader, the instructor can divide the group and assign one leader to every three or four students.

Taking a turn in team leading with a student group will help students with entry-to-practice competencies related to leadership in coordinating health care by

- providing practice in designing patient assignments based on factors such as acuity of the patients and nurses' experience and skill level;
- providing experience in supervising and evaluating the performance of other health-care providers; and
- providing experience with facilitating continuity of client care.

JACQUELINE MANN, MN, ACADEMIC COORDINATOR,
CENTRE FOR NURSING AND HEALTH STUDIES, ATHABASCA UNIVERSITY

From the Field   *Leading Rounds*

Rounds, traditionally defined as "a series of professional calls on hospital patients made by doctors or nurses" (Rounds, n.d.), can be adapted to a student-led learning activity.

Permission for the instructor and clinical group to visit and gather at the bedside must be obtained from the patient and unit or agency managers.

In preparation for leading the clinical group in a professional call or round with their patient or client, each student presents the patient to the clinical group, noting diagnosis, treatment, and plans for care.

Then, at the bedside, each student leads the round on this patient while the instructor and other members of the group observe the interaction and the environment. The round can include an introduction to the patient and a quick priority assessment such as ABCIOPS (A: airway, B: breathing, C: circulation, I: intake, O: output, P: pain and comfort, S: safety). As appropriate, the round may also include a chart review to highlight vital signs, procedures, and equipment being used.

Ensure that private space is available for the instructor and the group to debrief and exchange feedback after the round.

AMELIA CHAUVETTE, RN, BSCN, MSCN, THOMPSON RIVERS UNIVERSITY

Learning styles. Another strategy for clinical teachers to facilitate collaboration is to provide an opportunity for everyone in the group to complete an inventory of preferred learning styles. This is especially valuable at the beginning of a course. The process of teachers and students working together to discover and then share the ways in which they learn best can offer valuable reminders that everyone learns differently. The process can also remind teachers intentionally to implement a variety of different instructional approaches, not just those that they are familiar with or prefer themselves. A quick Google search will yield an abundance of inventories for preferred learning styles. Many of them are unsuitable because they are lengthy, must be purchased, or are restricted by copyright law. One inventory, the VAK/VARK questionnaire, is suitable and readily available for public use on the VARK (n.d.) website.

The VAK (Fleming & Mills, 1992; VARK, n.d.) model suggests that people prefer one of three styles of learning: visual, auditory (aural), or kinesthetic. Visual learners prefer movies, pictures, diagrams, displays, and handouts. They appreciate the opportunity to observe someone else complete a task or demonstrate it before they do it themselves. They work well from written directions. They might use phrases such as "show me." Auditory or aural learners prefer listening to spoken words or sounds. They value listening to instructions from experts. They work well from telephone or recorded directions. They might use phrases such as "tell me." Kinesthetic learners prefer physical experiences such as touching, feeling, holding, and doing. They are most comfortable learning tasks by stepping right in and trying to do what they are expected to do. They might use phrases such as "let me try." At different times and in different situations, people might prefer different ways of learning and combinations of learning styles.

An additional learning style, reading and writing, was later added to the VAK, which became the VARK (VARK, n.d.). Reading and writing learners prefer text-based information and materials. They are drawn to information presented in lists, manuals, textbooks, class notes, and PowerPoint lectures. They might use phrases such as "I read that."

A Strategy to Try ▶ *What's Your VARK?*

As a way of minimizing the hierarchy between teachers and students, try completing the VARK as a collaborative group activity early in the course. The VARK (visual, aural, reading and writing, kinesthetic) is an inventory of learning style preferences available for free at http://vark-learn.com/home/. Participants submit an online questionnaire and receive immediate feedback indicating the learning styles that they prefer. The site does not collect personal information.

Once you and your students have all completed the VARK, discuss the results. Some members of the group will prefer pictures and demonstrations (visual); some will prefer spoken words and recorded instructions (aural); some will prefer textbooks and PowerPoint lectures (reading and writing); and some will prefer touching and hands-on actions (kinesthetic). Most people value these different ways of learning but are particularly drawn to one or two. During the discussion of learning style preferences, ask for students' help in ensuring that your preferences do not dominate and that the student group shares responsibility for including a variety of different styles throughout the course.

CONCLUSION

In this chapter, we invited teachers to consider the idea of travelling with students as they journey toward their destination of becoming health-care professionals. Foundational knowledge from the discipline of education and the field of adult education can help clinical teachers to facilitate learning intentionally. Boyer's (1990) work articulating the scholarship inherent in teaching processes has encouraged educators to approach their work in new ways.

Teachers explore the everyday aspects of their practice through research studies and then disseminate their findings in peer-reviewed journals focused exclusively on education. Most health-care disciplines now have journals in which educators share research findings and best teaching practices.

Conceptual frameworks offer important guidance to teachers from a variety of disciplines. In health care, ideas from the invitational, constructivist, transformative, and Indigenous worldviews are particularly useful. Invitational views highlight welcoming learning environments that promote a climate of trust, respect, and optimism. A constructivist view emphasizes valuing what learners already know and builds instructional scaffolds to promote independence and extend existing knowledge. A transformative view stresses shifts in students' assumptions and gears learning experiences to triggering new insights and provoking critical reflection. Clinical learning activities that can provoke critical reflection include reflective journalling and case studies. An Indigenous view emphasizes the importance of "coming to" learning with an open mind and heart and adopting a holistic way of thinking that embraces interconnectivity with self, the land, and others.

Students who attend programs in postsecondary or higher education settings are considered adult learners. Theories and models from the field of adult education are based on the assumptions that adults bring life experiences to any learning event, that their learning needs are likely related to their changing social roles, and that they are motivated by internal rather than external factors. Adults learn best when addressing real-life problems, and they want to apply what they learn immediately. Foundational elements grounding most adult education theories are that adult learners value self-direction, experiential learning, and collaboration. Self-direction involves the ability to select, manage, and assess many of the activities needed for a learning experience. Experiential learning, or "learning by doing," means actually doing an activity and then reflecting analytically on the experience and imagining how the learning could apply beyond a particular setting. Collaboration involves sharing the responsibility for learning among groups of students and reducing hierarchical relationships between teachers and students.

In summary, in this chapter, we cast a spotlight on the notion that teaching can and should be viewed as a scholarly practice. The discipline of education offers clinical teachers a rich and abundant body of knowledge. Drawing from and contributing to this body of knowledge can be an exciting and fulfilling part of clinical teaching.

REFERENCES

About Education. (n.d.). *Pedagogy* [Definition]. http://k6educators.about.com/od/educationglossary/g/gpedagogy.htm

Alberta Regional Professional Development Consortium. (2018). *Weaving ways: Indigenous ways of knowing in classrooms and schools*. Alberta Education. http://empoweringthespirit.ca/wp-content/uploads/2018/09/Weaving-Ways-Introductory-Document-10-09.pdf

Anderson, J. R., & Tunney, N. M. (2014). The scholarship of teaching and learning in a physical therapy program. *New Directions for Teaching and Learning, 139*, 61–76. https://doi.org/10.1002/tl.20105

Association for Experiential Education. (n.d.) *What is experiential education?* [Fact sheet]. http://www.aee.org/ what-is-ee

Barkley, E., Cross, P., & Major, C. (2005). *Collaborative learning techniques: A handbook for college faculty*. Jossey-Bass.

Beckman, T., & Lee, M. (2009). Proposal for a collaborative approach to clinical teaching. *Mayo Clinic Proceedings, 84*(4), 339–344.

Boyer, E. L. (1990). *Scholarship reconsidered: Priorities of the professoriate*. Carnegie Foundation for the Advancement of Teaching. https://depts.washington.edu/gs630/Spring/Boyer.pdf

Brookfield, S. (1984). *Self-directed learning: From theory to practice*. Jossey-Bass.

Brookfield, S. (1986). *Understanding and facilitating adult learning*. Jossey-Bass.

Brookfield, S. (2012). *Teaching for critical thinking: Tools and techniques to help students question their assumptions*. Jossey-Bass.

Brookfield, S., & Preskill, S. (2005). *Discussion as a way of teaching: Tools and techniques for democratic classrooms*. Jossey-Bass.

Burrell, L. A. (2014). Integrating critical thinking strategies into nursing curricula. *Teaching and Learning in Nursing, 9*, 53–58. https://doi.org/10.1016/j.teln.2013.12.005

Canadian Association of Schools of Nursing (CASN). (2013). *CASN position statement on scholarship in nursing*. CASN. http://casn.ca/wp-content/uploads/2014/10/ScholarshipinNursingNov2013ENFINALmm.pdf

Carnegie Mellon. (n.d.). *Case studies* [Fact sheet]. Eberly Center: Teaching Excellence and Educational Innovation. https://www.cmu.edu/teaching/designteach/teach/instructionalstrategies/casestudies.html

Cash, P., & Tate, B. (2012). Fostering scholarship capacity: The experience of nurse educators. *The Canadian Journal for the Scholarship of Teaching and Learning, 3*(1), Art. 7. http://ir.lib.uwo.ca/cgi/viewcontent.cgi?article=1029&context=cjsotl_rcacea

Chan, C. (2009). *Assessment: Reflective journal* [Fact sheet]. Assessment Resources@ HKU, University of Hong Kong. http://ar.cetl.hku.hk/am_rj.htm#4

Chelliah, K., & Zain, N. (2016). Journal writing to promote reflective practice in medical imaging students. *Advanced Science Letters, 22*(12), 4561–4563. https://doi.org/10.1166/asl.2016.8221

Critical Thinking Community. (n.d.). *Our concept and definition of critical thinking* [Fact sheet]. http://www.criticalthinking.org/pages/our-concept-of-critical-thinking/411

Cull, I., Hancock, R. L. A., McKeown, S., Pidgeon, M., & Vedan, A. (2018). *Pulling together: A guide for front-line staff, student services, and advisors*. BCcampus. https://opentextbc.ca/indigenizationfrontlineworkers

Daloz, L. (2012). *Mentor: Guiding the journey of adult learners* (Rev. 2nd ed.). Jossey-Bass.

Dewey, J. (1938). *Experience and education*. Macmillan.

Douglass, C., & Morris, S. (2014). Student perspectives on self-directed learning. *Journal of the Scholarship of Teaching and Learning, 14*(1), 13–25.

Duncan, S., Mahara, S., & Holmes, V. (2014). Confronting the social mandate for nursing scholarship—One school of nursing's journey. *Quality Advancement in Nursing Education, 1*(1), Art. 2. http://qane-afi.casn.ca/cgi/viewcontent.cgi?article=1018&context=journal

Educate [Definition]. (n.d.). In *Oxford dictionary*. http://www.oxforddictionaries.com/definition/english/pedagogy

Ekelin, M., Kvist, L., Thies-Lagergren, L. & Persson, E. (2021). Clinical supervisors' experiences of midwifery students' reflective writing: A process for mutual professional growth. *Reflective Practice, 22*(1), 101–114. https://doi.org/10.1080/14623943.2020.1854211

First Nations Education Steering Committee. (n.d.). *First Peoples principles of learning* [Fact sheet]. https://firstpeoplesprinciplesoflearning.wordpress.com/background-and-current-context/

Fleming, N. D., & Mills, C. (1992). Not another inventory, rather a catalyst for reflection. *To Improve the Academy, 11*, 137–155. http://vark-learn.com/wp-content/uploads/2014/08/not_another_inventory.pdf

Gaberson, K., Oermann, M., & Shellenbarger, T. (2015). Case method, case study, and grand rounds. In *Clinical teaching strategies in nursing* (4th ed., pp. 237–254). Springer.

Ganzer, C., & Zauderer, C. (2013). Structured learning and self-reflection: Strategies to decrease anxiety in the psychiatric mental health clinical nursing experience. *Nursing Education Perspectives, 34*(4), 244–247. https://doi.org/10.5480/1536-5026-34.4.244

Garrity, M. (2013). Developing nursing leadership skills through reflective journaling: A nursing professor's personal reflection. *Reflective Practice, 14*(1), 118–130. https://doi.org/10.1080/14623943.2012.732940

Glassick, C. E. (2000). Boyer's expanded definitions of scholarship, the standards for assessing scholarship, and the elusiveness of the scholarship of teaching. *Academic Medicine, 75*(9), 877–880.

Glassick, C. E., Huber, M. T., & Maeroff, G. I. (1997). *Scholarship assessed: Evaluation of the Professoriate*. Jossey-Bass.

Gubbins, p. (2014). An opportunity for academic faculty members in pharmacy and other health professions to develop a program of scholarship. *International Journal of Scholarship in Teaching and Learning, 8*(1), Art. 3. http://digitalcommons. georgiasouthern.edu/cgi/viewcontent.cgi?article=1417&context=ij-sotl

Guglielmino, L. (2014). Self-directed learning for the 21st century—What research says. *International Journal of Self-Directed Learning, 1*(7), No. 2 [Blog]. http:// www.p21.org/ news-events/p21blog/1472

Hagler, D., White, B., & Morris, B. (2011). Cognitive tools as a scaffold for faculty during curriculum redesign. *Journal of Nursing Education, 50*(7), 417–422. https://doi.org/10.3928/01484834-20110214-03

Hansson, S. O. (2019). Critical thinking. *Theoria, 85*, 3–7. https://doi.org/10.1111/ theo.12179. https://onlinelibrary.wiley.com/doi/epdf/10.1111/theo.12179

Imel, S. (1991). *Collaborative learning in adult education* (ERIC Digest No. 113). ERIC. http://files.eric.ed.gov/fulltext/ED334469.pdf

International Society for Self-Directed Learning. (n.d.). *About us* [Webpage]. https:// www.sdlglobal.com/about-us

Jacobson, M., & Ruddy, M. (2004). *Open to outcome: A practical guide for facilitating and teaching experiential reflection.* Wood 'N' Barnes.

Jarvis, M., & Baloyi, O. (2020). Scaffolding in reflective journaling: A means to develop higher order thinking skills in undergraduate learners. *International Journal of Africa Nursing Sciences, 12*, Art. 100195. https://doi.org/10.1016/j. ijans.2020.100195

King, A. (1993). From sage on the stage to guide on the side. *College Teaching, 41*(1), 30–35.

Knowles, M. (1975). *Self-directed learning: A guide for learners and teachers.* Association Press.

Knowles, M. (1980). *The modern practice of adult education: From pedagogy to andragogy* (2nd ed.). Cambridge Books.

Knowles, M. (1984). *Andragogy in action.* Jossey-Bass.

Kohn, A. (2012). The case against grades. *The Education Digest, 77*(5), 8–16.

Kolb, D. A. (1984). *Experiential learning: Experience as the source of learning and development.* Prentice-Hall.

Kolb, D. A., & Fry, R. (1975). Toward an applied theory of experiential learning. In C. Cooper (Ed.), *Theories of group process* (pp. 33–58). John Wiley.

Kurczek, J., & Johnson, J. (2014). The student as teacher: Reflections on collaborative learning in a senior seminar. *Journal of Undergraduate Neuroscience Education, 12*(2), A93–A99.

Lasater, K., & Nielsen, A. (2009). Reflective journaling for clinical judgment development and evaluation. *Journal of Nursing Education, 48*(1), 40–44. https:// doi.org/10.3928/01484834-20090101-06

Melrose, S. (2017). Pass/fail and discretionary grading: A snapshot of their influences on learning. *Open Journal of Nursing, 7*, 185–192. http://www.scirp.org/ journal/ojn

Melrose, S., Park, C., & Perry, B. (2013). *Teaching health professionals online.* Athabasca University Press. https://doi.org/10.15215/aupress/ 9781927356654.01

MERLOT Health Sciences. (n.d.). *MERLOT Health Sciences* [Website]. California State University. http://healthsciences.merlot.org/

Mezirow, J. (1978). Perspective transformation. *Adult Education Quarterly, 28*(2), 100–109. https://doi.org/10.1177/074171367802800202

Mezirow, J. (1981). A critical theory of adult learning and education. *Adult Education Quarterly, 32,* 3–23.

Mezirow, J. (1997). Transformative learning: Theory to practice. *New Directions for Adult and Continuing Education, 74,* 5–12.

Mezirow, J. (2009). An overview on transformative learning. In K. Illeris (Ed.), *Contemporary theories of learning: Learning theorists in their own words* (pp. 90–105). Routledge.

Moon, J. (2004). *A handbook of reflective and experiential learning: Theory and practice.* Routledge-Farmer.

Morgan, K., & Brooks, D. W. (2012). Investigating a method of scaffolding student-designed experiments. *Journal of Science Education and Technology, 21*(4), 513–522. https://doi.org/10.1007/s10956-011-9343-y

Nevers, S., & Melrose, S. (2016). Posing questions to support and challenge: A guide for mentoring staff. *Internet Journal of Allied Health Sciences and Practice, 14*(3), Art. 2. https://nsuworks.nova.edu/ijahsp/vol14/iss3/2/

Oermann, M. (2015). Becoming a scholar in nursing education. In M. Oermann (Ed.), *Teaching in nursing and role of the educator: The complete guide to best practice in teaching, evaluation, and curriculum development.* Springer.

Palmer, P. J. (1983/1993). *To know as we are known: Education as a spiritual journey.* Harper.

Palmer, P. J. (1998). *The courage to teach: Exploring the inner landscape of a teacher's life.* Jossey-Bass.

Palmer, p. (2007). *The courage to teach: Exploring the inner landscape of a teacher's life.* 10th anniversary ed. Jossey-Bass.

Paul, R., & Elder, L. (2007). Critical thinking: The art of Socratic questioning. *Journal of Developmental Education, 31*(1), 36–37.

Piaget, J. (1972). *Psychology and epistemology: Toward a theory of knowledge.* Penguin.

Popil, I. (2011). Promotion of critical thinking by using case studies as teaching method. *Nurse Education Today, 31,* 204–207. https://doi.org/10.1016/ j.nedt.2010.06.002

Purkey, W. (1992). An introduction to invitational theory. *Journal of Invitational Theory and Practice, 1*(1), 5–15.

Ross, C., Mahal, K., Chinnapen, Y., Kolar, M., & Woodman, K. (2014). Evaluation of nursing students' work experience through the use of reflective journals. *Mental Health Practice, 17*(6), 21–27.

Rounds [Definition 1]. (n.d.). In *Merriam-Webster medical dictionary online.* http:// www.merriam-webster.com/medical/rounds

Rowles, C. J. (2012). Strategies to promote critical thinking and active learning. In D. Billings & J. Halstead (Eds.), *Teaching in nursing: A guide for faculty* (4th ed.) (pp. 258–280). Saunders.

Sanders, D., & Welk, D. S. (2005). Strategies to scaffold student learning: Applying Vygotsky's zone of proximal development. *Nurse Educator, 30*(5), 203–207.

Shaw, G. B. (n.d.). *George Bernard Shaw quotes.* https://www.quotes.net/quote/387

Shaw, G. B. (1908). *Getting married* [Play]. http://www.gutenberg.org/ebooks/5604

Shulman, L. S. (1998). *Course anatomy: The dissection and analysis of knowledge through teaching.* American Association of Higher Education. http://www.vet.utk.edu/enhancement/pdf/future2.pdf

Snively, G., & Williams, W. (2016). *Knowing home: Braiding Indigenous science with Western science.* University of Victoria. https://pressbooks.bccampus.ca/knowinghome/

Tomey, A. M. (2003). Learning with cases. *The Journal of Continuing Education in Nursing, 34*(1), 34–38.

Turner, p. (2005). Critical thinking in nursing education and practice as defined in the literature. *Nursing Education Perspectives, 26*(5), 272–277.

VARK. (n.d.). *Visual aural read/write kinesthetic VARK: A guide to learning styles* [Webpage]. http://vark-learn.com/home/

Vygotsky, L. S. (1978). *Mind and society: The development of higher psychological processes.* Harvard University Press.

Waldo, N., & Hermanns, M. (2009). Journaling unlocks fears in clinical practice. *RN, 72*(5), 26–31.

White, C. (2010). Pass-fail grading: Laying the foundation for self-regulated learning. *Advances in Health Sciences Education, 15*(4), 469–477.

Woodley, L. (2015). Clinical teaching in nursing. In M. Oermann (Ed.), *Teaching in nursing and role of the educator: The complete guide to best practice in teaching, evaluation, and curriculum development.* Springer.

Zygmont, D., & Moore Schaefer, K. (2006). Assessing the critical thinking skills of faculty: What do the findings mean for nursing education? *Nursing Education Perspectives, 27*(5), 260–268.

2

Where Do I Fit In?

Articulating a Personal Philosophy

If we possess our why of life we can put up with almost any how.
FRIEDRICH NIETZSCHE (1889/1968, P. 23)

Teachers bring unique philosophies and viewpoints to their interactions with students. Some of these views are more obvious than others. For example, some teachers might state that they choose teaching to help and support new members of their profession. Others might note that involvement with learners is an expected job requirement. Taking the time to reflect on and begin to articulate a personal philosophy of teaching can help teachers to understand why they approach their practice in particular ways and how their individual views fit with "big picture" educational issues. Understanding *why* a teaching approach or action might be advantageous before deciding *what* content to implement or *how* to deliver that content helps teachers to think critically about their practice.

Any philosophy or expression of beliefs can evolve and grow over time. As teachers strengthen their theoretical knowledge and gain practical experience, their personal teaching philosophy will also change. Although it can seem daunting to try to put beliefs into words, initiating a working teaching philosophy statement and then adding to it throughout your career can support teachers in becoming more engaged, competent, and scholarly

(Chism, 1998; Goodyear & Allchin, 1998; Owens et al., 2014; Ratnapradipa & Adams, 2012; Schönwetter et al., 2002; Yeom et al., 2018).

For clinical teachers who seek to identify where they fit in and how best to articulate a personal philosophy of teaching, established philosophical perspectives from the field of adult education offer important direction. Liberal, behaviourist, progressive, humanist, and radical perspectives are traditionally considered foundational. Each of these overarching perspectives brings different underlying assumptions about human nature, the purpose of education, the role of the educator, and the role of the learner. Perspectives specific to teaching, such as transmission, apprenticeship, developmental, nurturing, and social reform perspectives, provide more explicit guidance for those in higher education. In this chapter, we provide a primer on key adult educational philosophies and discuss the process of articulating a personal teaching philosophy statement.

A PRIMER ON KEY ADULT EDUCATION PHILOSOPHIES

Five Key Adult Education Philosophies

An adult education philosophy or perspective is the categorization of an individual's beliefs, values, and attitudes regarding education. In this section, we present Elias and Merriam's (1995) seminal work identifying the five key adult education philosophies of liberal, behaviourist, progressive, humanist, and radical perspectives.

A *liberal* perspective emphasizes the development of intellectual abilities. Liberal education is related to liberal arts, not to liberal political views. A liberal arts education provides general knowledge with an emphasis on reasoning and judgment instead of professional, vocational, or technical skills (Liberal arts education, n.d.). A liberal education promotes theoretical thinking and stresses philosophy, religion, and the humanities over science.

Liberal teachers are experts who transmit knowledge, direct the learning process with authority, and emphasize organized knowledge. Teachers play a prominent role in this philosophy and have a variety of intellectual interests. Teaching methods focus on lectures, readings, study groups, and discussions. Socrates, Plato, and Jean Piaget are considered liberal teachers.

A *behaviourist* perspective emphasizes skill acquisition. Behaviourist education conditions and shapes individuals through clearly defined purposes and learning objectives. Heavy emphasis is placed on assessing and evaluating whether behaviours taught have been learned.

Behaviourist teachers manage learning environments in ways that promote the learning of expected and desired behaviours. Although teachers reinforce or positively acknowledge students when they succeed, both teachers and students are accountable for learning success. Mastery learning and standards-based education are often framed from a behaviourist perspective. Teaching methods include programmed instruction, contract learning, and computer-guided instruction. Ivan Pavlov, Burrhus Frederic Skinner, and John Watson made significant contributions to this perspective.

A *progressive* perspective emphasizes an experiential, problem-solving approach to learning. Progressive education liberates learners and equips them to solve problems and apply practical knowledge. Students learn by doing, inquiring, being involved in the community, and responding to real-life problems. Progressive thinking is grounded in five principles. First, education is viewed as a lifelong process and not one restricted to formal classroom instruction. Second, learners can learn more than their immediate interests. Third, they value diverse instructional methodologies. Fourth, teacher-learner relationships are interactive and reciprocal. Fifth, education prepares learners to change society.

Teaching methods include the scientific method, problem-based learning, and cooperative learning. Proponents of this perspective include John Dewey, Francis Parker, and Edward Lindeman.

A *humanist* perspective underscores personal growth and development. Humanistic education supports learners to become fully functional and self-actualized. Humanists believe that individuals are autonomous and have unlimited potential that should be nurtured. They also believe that individuals have a responsibility to humanity.

Learners are viewed as highly motivated, self-directed, and responsible for their own learning. Humanist teachers facilitate and partner with students rather than manage or direct their learning. "Humanist adult educators are concerned with the development of the whole person with a special emphasis upon the emotional and affective dimensions of the personality" (Elias & Merriam, 1995, p. 109).

Table 1—Philosophies of Adult Education

	LIBERAL	BEHAVIOURIST
Purpose of education	Develop intellectual abilities	Emphasize skill acquisition
View of learner	Always a learner Seeks knowledge rather than information	Needs to practise new behaviour Strong environmental influence on learning
Role of teacher	Experts who transmit knowledge Direct the learning process	Manage, control, and positively reinforce Predict and direct learning outcomes
Methods	Lectures, readings, discussion groups	Programmed instruction, computer-assisted learning
Key words	Learning for its own sake Classical, traditional	Stimulus-response Behaviour modification Learning objectives and evaluation of those objectives
Authors	Socrates, Plato, Piaget	Pavlov, Skinner, Watson
Examples	University or college lectures	CPR certification and renewal

Note. Adapted from Elias and Merriam (1980) and Zinn (1983, 1994, 1998).

PROGRESSIVE	HUMANIST	RADICAL
Equip learners with practical knowledge and problem-solving skills	Enhance personal growth, development	Promote fundamental social, political, and economic changes in society
Learn by doing, experimenting, and working with real-life problems	Motivated, self-directed, responsible Learners have unlimited potential	Equal to the teacher within the learning process
Organize, establish, and guide interactive reciprocal relationships with learners	Facilitate, support, and partner Attentive to emotional and affective issues	Coordinates and suggests but does not determine direction of learning
Problem-based learning, cooperative learning	Team teaching, group tasks, individualized learning	Group identifies problems to solve, discussion groups
Based on experience Democratic principles Problem solving	Self-actualization, cooperation, group work, self-direction	Raising of awareness of social problems Social action Non-compulsory learning activities
Dewey, Parker, Lindeman	Rogers, Maslow, Knowles	Friere, Illich, Holt
Problem-based health-care programs	Clinical pre-and post-conferences	Literacy training

Teaching methods include team teaching, group tasks, group discussion, and individualized learning. Theories developed by Carl Rogers, Abraham Maslow, and Malcolm Knowles ground this perspective.

A *radical* perspective highlights social, political, and economic change through education. Rather than working within existing norms and structures, radical education often occurs outside mainstream adult and higher education programs. Radical educationalists value non-compulsory and informal learning activities.

Radical teachers coordinate, make suggestions, and partner with learners. They do not direct the learning process. Teaching methods include exposure to the media and real-life situations. Paulo Freire, Ivan Illich, and John Holt are well-known radical thinkers.

A Strategy to Try ▶ *My Favourite Philosophies*
Review each of the boxes in Table 1, *Philosophies of Adult Education*. Put a checkmark beside any comments in the boxes that seem to resonate for you. Do your checkmarks fall into one or two favourite philosophies? Do some philosophies seem to fit you better than others?

PHILOSOPHY OF ADULT EDUCATION INVENTORY

Building upon the five key adult education philosophies of liberal, behaviourist, progressive, humanist, and radical described above, Lorraine Zinn (1983, 1994, 1998) developed a classic questionnaire that teachers can use to help identify the perspective(s) to which they are most drawn. The Philosophy of Adult Education Inventory (PAEI) is available for free on the LabR Learning Resources webpage. To complete the questionnaire, respond to each inventory question by selecting from a scale ranging from *Strongly Disagree* to *Strongly Agree*. Once you have submitted your responses, an inventory of results will be emailed to you. Most teachers are drawn to more than just one philosophical perspective.

FIVE PERSPECTIVES ON TEACHING ADULTS

The general philosophies of education can be contrasted with the specific
ideas among teachers about what they do and would like to do in their
day-to-day practice. A teaching perspective is an interrelated set of beliefs
and intentions that justifies and directs teachers' actions (Pratt, 1998).
Teaching perspectives are more than teaching styles. They "determine our
roles and idealized self-images as teachers as well as the basis for reflecting on practice" (Pratt, 1998, p. 35). The seminal work of Pratt et al. (2001)
examining teachers' actions, intentions, and beliefs describes five perspectives on teaching: transmission, apprenticeship, developmental, nurturing,
and social reform.

Transmission teachers strive for effective delivery of content. They are
masters of subject matter. They set high standards for achievement and
direct students to useful resources. They provide reviews, summaries, and
objective methods of assessing learning. They clarify misunderstandings,
answer questions, and correct errors.

Apprenticeship teachers model ways of being. They "reveal the inner
workings of skilled performance and must now translate it into accessible
language and an ordered set of tasks" (Pratt & Collins, n.d., p. 2). They guide
students from simple to more complex activities and gradually withdraw
as learners assume more responsibility for their learning.

Developmental teachers cultivate ways of thinking. They believe that
teaching is planned and focused from the learner's point of view. They
seek to understand how learners are thinking and reasoning and then try
to support them to achieve more sophisticated ways of comprehending
content. They provide meaningful examples and use questions to move
learners from simple to more complex ways of thinking.

Nurturing teachers facilitate self-efficacy. They have confidence in their students. They believe that their students succeed because of their own efforts and abilities, not because of the benevolence of a teacher. They teach "from the heart as well as the head" (Pratt & Collins, n.d., p. 4).

Social reform teachers seek a better society. They endeavour to make significant changes at the societal level. They are interested in the values and ideologies that are part of everyday practice.

TEACHING PERSPECTIVES INVENTORY

Another highly regarded inventory to help teachers articulate their own philosophy of teaching is the Teaching Perspectives Inventory (TPI) developed by University of British Columbia professor Daniel Pratt and associates (Pratt, 1998; Pratt & Collins, n.d.). The TPI is available for free on the Teaching Perspectives Inventory website. Once you have submitted your responses, a profile of results will be emailed to you. This profile reflects your dominant, backup, and recessive perspectives. Further instructions for interpreting and understanding your profile are posted on the website.

A Strategy to Try ▶ *Try the Teaching Perspectives Inventory*
Visit the Teaching Perspectives Inventory website (http://www.teaching-perspectives.com/tpi/) and complete the inventory. Review your profile in relation to the instructions on the "Reflecting on Results" tab. Most teachers embrace aspects of all five perspectives. However, the TPI will identify dominant, backup, and recessive perspectives that are unique to you. Keep a record of your profile and complete the inventory again from time to time to observe any changes.

A teaching philosophy includes reflections on our beliefs about teaching and how we act on those beliefs in our everyday teaching practice. Although senior clinical instructors might have developed and established their personal philosophies, new teachers might not yet have had such opportunities.

During orientation, take some time to reflect on the question "What is my philosophy of teaching?" Begin your reflection by thinking about your hopes when you first applied for a teaching position. Write down your thoughts and be sure to revisit and revise your views at the start and end of each term you teach.

Putting our beliefs into words is an important first step in the ongoing process of establishing a philosophy of teaching. Teaching is different from bedside nursing. Understanding our philosophy can help us to create balance during times when teaching tasks such as client assessment seem to override more complex teaching topics such as empathy. It can also help when new areas of expertise and responsibility seem to be overwhelming.

KARA SEALOCK, RN EDD CNCC(C), NURSING PRACTICE INSTRUCTOR, FACULTY OF NURSING, UNIVERSITY OF CALGARY

THE PROCESS OF ARTICULATING A PERSONAL TEACHING PHILOSOPHY STATEMENT

What Is a Teaching Philosophy Statement?

Articulating a personal philosophy of teaching is increasingly important among those who teach in health education (Ratnapradipa & Adams, 2012), pharmacy (Medina & Draugalis, 2013), physiology (Kearns & Sullivan, 2011), social work (Owens et al., 2014), recreational therapy (Stevens et al., 2012), nursing (Horsfall et al., 2012; Spurr et al., 2010), and other health disciplines. A teaching philosophy or teaching philosophy statement puts into words what we believe about the general purpose of teaching, how students learn, how instructors can best intervene throughout the process of learning, and how our beliefs will translate into actions (Chism, 1998; Goodyear & Allchin, 1998; Grundman, 2006).

A seminal definition is that a teaching philosophy statement is "a systematic and critical rationale that focuses on the important components defining effective teaching and learning in a particular discipline and/or institutional context" (Schönwetter et al., 2002, p. 84). Crafting a teaching philosophy statement is expected to be an ongoing reflective process that articulates where teachers are now and their goals for the future (Beatty et al., 2009). It should be revised and revisited frequently (Chism, 1998). Even when not formally articulated, teaching philosophies influence how teachers plan learning activities, interact with students, and even react to student misconduct (Coughlin, 2014).

The content of a teaching philosophy statement will be very different for each individual. According to Chism (1998, p. 1), it should be written in the first person, not exceed two pages in length, avoid technical terms, incorporate metaphors, and "be reflective and personal." Mentioning the names of educational scholars might be valuable, but a substantive literature review is not usually included (University of Toronto, n.d.). Teaching statements are meant to be viewed by others, so starting one with a brief self-introduction can be useful.

Some teachers might choose to start their reflections by reminiscing about their own experiences as learners. Thinking about teachers who had positive or negative influences can provide valuable insights. Similarly, beginning the reflective process by musing on an inspirational quotation or image can provide some insight. Recalling why you first went into teaching can also be valuable. The decision to include these reflections is optional. A Google search using terms such as "writing a teaching philosophy statement" or "examples of a teaching philosophy statement" will yield a plethora of examples of how other educators have crafted their statements. Similarly, asking colleagues about their teaching philosophies can provide inspiration.

Generally, four common areas of focus are addressed in today's teaching philosophy statements (Owens et al., 2014):

1. conceptualization of how learning occurs
2. conceptualization of an effective teaching and learning environment
3. expectations of the teacher-student relationship
4. student assessment and assessment of learning goals

O'Neal et al. (2007, p. 2) propose a concrete and manageable way to approach these "big picture" areas of focus. To get started on a statement of one's teaching philosophy, they suggest answering the following questions and then assembling the answers into a holistic and personalized essay.

- Why do you teach?
- What do you believe or value about teaching and student learning?
- If you had to choose a metaphor for teaching/learning, what would it be?
- How do your research and disciplinary context influence your teaching?
- How do your identity/background and your students' identities/backgrounds affect teaching and learning in your classes?
- How do you take into account differences in learning styles in your teaching?
- What is your approach to evaluating and assessing students?

A Strategy to Try ▶ *Getting Started on a Teaching Philosophy Statement*
Jot down your answers to this list of questions. Although you will likely rewrite and polish your comments when assembling your responses into a document to be shared with others, your first responses might be the heart of your beliefs about teaching.

Finally, include a section on goals and how you are implementing and evaluating them. Comment on the kind of educator whom you hope to be in 5 or 10 years. Which specific actions are you taking to achieve your goals? Some teachers might include brief mentions of teaching materials that they have created or revised. However, a teaching philosophy statement is not a curriculum vitae; it is a developing illustration of your reflections and aspirations at a particular time.

The Centre for Teaching Support and Innovation at the University of Toronto (n.d.) identifies the following pitfalls to avoid when writing a teaching philosophy statement:

- *Too general*—limited expressions of your own beliefs, experiences, and circumstances
- *Not reflective*—lists techniques and approaches rather than describes how they have contributed to your beliefs
- *Too negative*—dwells on negatives without a balance of positives
- *Too clichéd*—expresses a belief in a popular or contemporary approach to teaching without noting how that approach is integrated into your teaching
- *Too few examples*—lacks examples of what you are doing and how you know whether it is effective or not

Once you have started a teaching philosophy statement, plan to add to it regularly and systematically. If you are applying for teaching positions at universities, a teaching philosophy statement is often a required part of job and promotion applications. Lang (2010, p. 2) encourages teachers to write a statement "that doesn't sound like [those of] everybody else." He invites teachers to picture a student walking into their class and then imagine in what way the student will be different at the end of the course. Lang suggests that, "as soon as you describe your teaching objectives, tell a story about how your objectives played out . . . [as] an enlightening moment . . . or even a moment of failure" (p. 15). No two teaching philosophy statements will be or should be alike. Although they are expected to be readable and well organized, there are no right or wrong processes for creating these working documents.

A Strategy to Try ▶ *Share Your Teaching Philosophy Statement*
Develop a two-page document from the notes and ideas that you have gathered in reading about established philosophies of adult education and the process of articulating a teaching philosophy statement. Organize your points and be sure to balance your narrative with personal experiences or anecdotes. Ask a respected colleague or mentor to look at your statement and offer feedback. Think about sharing your statement with your students. If you have a professional website, then consider posting your teaching philosophy statement on it.

CONCLUSION

In this chapter, we presented a primer on liberal, behaviourist, progressive, humanist, and radical philosophical perspectives from the field of adult education. These well-known and enduring perspectives offer useful foundational knowledge to teachers as they reflect on their own beliefs about human nature, the purpose of education, the role of the educator, and the role of the learner. Each of these perspectives paints a different picture of teachers. A liberal perspective views teachers as experts; a behaviourist perspective views them as managers; a progressive perspective views them as partners; a humanist perspective views them as supporters; and a radical perspective views teachers as coordinators. The Philosophy of Adult Education Inventory is a free questionnaire that teachers can complete for help in understanding to which philosophical perspectives they are most drawn. The PAEI is available at http://www.labr.net/paei/paei.html.

We discussed five perspectives specific to teaching in higher education: transmission, apprenticeship, developmental, nurturing, and social reform perspectives. Each casts a spotlight on specific aspects of teachers' roles in different ways. Transmission teachers are masters of subject matter; apprenticeship teachers model ways of being; developmental teachers cultivate ways of thinking; nurturing teachers facilitate self-efficacy; and social reform teachers seek to change society. The Teaching Perspectives Inventory is another free questionnaire that teachers can complete to gain a deeper understanding of which perspectives resonate with them. The TPI is available at http://www.teachingperspectives.com/tpi/.

The process of articulating a personal statement of teaching philosophy is seldom straightforward. We have provided guidance with suggestions such as writing in the first person, including metaphors, and reflecting on personally meaningful stories. Most teaching philosophy statements include your beliefs about how learning occurs, what an effective teaching and learning environment looks like, what you expect from your teacher-student relationships, and your views on assessment. Teaching philosophy statements are working documents that should be revised frequently and shared with others. They can be required for job and promotion applications at universities.

In sum, understanding why teachers do what they do begins with reviewing established educational philosophies. This understanding provides a foundation for the ongoing process of creating a reflective and personal philosophy, one that is unique to you.

REFERENCES

Beatty, J., Leigh, J., & Dean, K. (2009). Finding our roots: An exercise for creating a personal teaching philosophy statement. *Journal of Management Education, 33*, 115–130.

Chism, N. V. N. (1998). Developing a philosophy of teaching statement. *Essays on Teaching Excellence: Toward the Best in the Academy, 9*(3), 1–3. Professional and Organizational Development Network in Higher Education.

Coughlin, D. (2014). Enhancing your teaching experience: Developing your teaching philosophy, course syllabus, and teaching portfolio. *The Industrial-Organizational Psychologist, 52*(2), 94–99.

Elias, J. L., & Merriam, S.B. (1980). *Philosophical foundations of adult education.* Krieger.

Elias, J. L., & Merriam, S. B. (1995). *Philosophical foundations of adult education* (2nd ed.). Krieger.

Goodyear, G. E., & Allchin, D. (1998). Statement of teaching philosophy. *To Improve the Academy, 17*, 103–122.

Grundman, H. (2006). Writing a teaching philosophy statement. *Notices of the American Mathematical Society AMS, 53*, 1329–1333.

Horsfall, J., Cleary, M., & Hunt, G. (2012). Developing a pedagogy for nursing teaching-learning. *Nurse Education Today, 32*(8), 930–933. https://doi.org/10.1016/j.nedt.2011.10.022

Kearns, K., & Sullivan, C. (2011). Resources and practices to help graduate students and postdoctoral fellows write statements of teaching philosophy. *Advances in Physiology Education, 35*, 136–145.

Lang, J. (2010). 4 steps to a memorable teaching philosophy [Advice]. *The Chronicle of Higher Education.* http://chronicle.com/article/ 4-Steps-to-a-Memorable/124199/?sid=ja&utm_source=ja&utm_medium=en

Liberal arts education. (n.d.). In *Merriam-Webster online.* http://www.merriam-webster.com/dictionary/liberal%20arts

Medina, M., & Draugalis, J. (2013). Writing a teaching philosophy: An evidence-based approach. *American Journal of Health-System Pharmacy, 70*(3), 191–193. https://doi.org/10.2146/ajhp120418

Nietzsche, F. (1968). *Twilight of the idols* (R.J. Hollingdale, Trans.). Penguin. (Original work published 1889.)

O'Neal, C., Meizlish, D., & Kaplan, M. (2007). Writing a statement of teaching philosophy for the academic job search. CRLT Occasional Paper 23 (pp.1–8), Ann Arbor, MI: University of Michigan Center for Research on Learning and Teaching. http://www.crlt.umich.edu/sites/default/files/resource_files/CRLT_no23.pdf

Owens, L., Miller, J., & Owens, E. (2014). Activating a teaching philosophy in social work education: Articulation, implementation, and evaluation. *Journal of Teaching in Social Work, 34*(3), 332–345. https://doi.org/10.1080/08841233.2014.907597

Pratt, D. D. (1998). *Five perspectives on teaching in adult and higher education*. Krieger.

Pratt, D., & Collins, J. (n.d.). *Teaching perspectives inventory*. http://www.teaching perspectives.com/tpi/

Pratt, D., Collins, J., & Selinger, S. (2001). *Development and use of the Teaching Perspectives Inventory (TPI)*. Paper presented at the 2001 American Association of Educational Researchers Annual Meeting, Seattle, WA. https://faculty commons.macewan.ca/wp-content/uploads/TPI-online-resource.pdf

Ratnapradipa, D., & Adams, T. (2012). Framing the teaching philosophy statement for health educators: What it includes and how it can inform professional development. *The Health Educator, 44*(1), 37–42.

Schönwetter, D., Sokal, L., Friesen, M., & Taylor, L. (2002). Teaching philosophies reconsidered: A conceptual model for the development and evaluation of teaching philosophy statements. *International Journal for Academic Development, 7*(1), 83–97.

Spurr, S., Bally, J., & Ferguson, L. (2010). A framework for clinical teaching: A passion centered philosophy. *Nurse Education in Practice, 10*(6), 349–354. https://doi.org/10.1016/j.nepr.2010.05.002

Stevens, C., Schneider, P. P., & Johnson, C. W. (2012). Preparing students to write a professional philosophy of recreation paper. *Schole: A Journal of Leisure Studies and Recreation Education, 27*(2), 43–56.

University of Toronto. (n.d.). *Writing a statement of teaching philosophy* [Tip sheet]. Centre for Teaching Support and Innovation. http://www.teaching.utoronto. ca/topics/documenting-teaching/s-t-p.htm

Yeom, Y., Miller, M., & Delp, R. (2018). Constructing a teaching philosophy: Aligning beliefs, theories, and practice. *Teaching and Learning in Nursing, 13*, 131–134. https://doi.org/10.1016/j.teln.2018.01.004

Zinn, L. (1983). Development of a valid and reliable instrument for adult educators to identify a personal philosophy of adult education. *Dissertation Abstracts International, 44*, 1667A–1668A.

Zinn, L. (1994). *Philosophy of adult education inventory* (Rev. ed.). Lifelong Learning Options.

Zinn, L. (1998). Identifying your philosophical orientation. In M. W. Galbraith (Ed.), *Adult learning methods* (2nd ed., pp. 37–72). Krieger. http://www.labr.net/ apps/paei/zinn.pdf

3

The Clinical Learning Environment

Encouragement after censure is as the sun after a shower.
JOHANN WOLFGANG VON GOETHE (1853/2013, P. 55)

Today's clinical learning environments can seem overwhelming. Learners, instructors, and staff members all face extraordinary challenges in healthcare workplaces. Students can be recent high school graduates, adult learners supporting families, or newcomers to the country who continue to work on their language and literacy skills. Common concerns are high costs of tuition, which result in unmanageable debt, and competition to achieve top marks. Many students travel significant distances to the clinical site and balance heavy study commitments.

Similarly, instructors are often employed only on a sessional or contract basis. They also balance work and family obligations that are separate from the clinical learning environment. As well, professional staff members at a clinical site, ultimately responsible for client safety and care, are frequently employed on a contract basis and might work at several different facilities. At times, they might view learners as an additional burden rather than an opportunity for professional development. Non-professional staff might find themselves assisting learners.

Creating a learning community among learners, teachers, and staff cannot be left to chance. The complex social context of the current clinical learning environment makes intentional teaching approaches essential, approaches grounded in an understanding of how learning occurs for students. In this chapter, we discuss the clinical learning environment, who the teachers are, and who the students are. We provide creative and easy-to-implement strategies that offer practical guidance to instructors for managing the everyday occurrences faced by clinical teachers in this unique "classroom."

PICTURE OF THE CLINICAL LEARNING ENVIRONMENT

Students in health-care education programs at universities complete practicums in a clinical learning environment in addition to attending academic classes. Clinical practicums are considered essential to professional competence in most health-based professions. For example, clinical practicums are viewed as essential to the curriculum by programs in medicine (Ruesseler & Obertacke, 2011), nursing (Courtney-Pratt et al., 2011), pharmacy (Krueger, 2013), physical therapy (Buccieri et al., 2013; McCallum et al., 2013), occupational therapy (Rodger et al., 2011), dietetics (Dietitians of Canada, n.d.), radiation therapy (Leaver, 2012), paramedic training (McCall et al., 2009), and dental hygiene (Paulis, 2011). Internationally, clinical practicum placements for students in these and other health-care disciplines are in markedly short supply. Available placements might be in programs offering care only to seriously ill clients, might be inundated with learners from the health disciplines, and might be experiencing budget cuts and staff shortages (Brown et al., 2011; Roger et al., 2008).

The real-world learning environment in which students in the health professions complete their clinical practicums is an "interactive network of forces" (Dunn & Burnett, 1995) rich in opportunities for learners to transfer theory to practice. Sequences of learning activities in unpredictable clinical environments can be more difficult to plan and structure than in traditional classroom environments. Both planned and unplanned experiences must be taken into account.

PLANNED EXPERIENCES

Following direction from a *curriculum* is a widely used planned learning experience in the clinical learning environment of any professional health-care program. At the curricular level, clinical practicums are usually arranged before students are granted admission to their programs of study. A curriculum is the range of courses and experiences that a learner must complete successfully in order to graduate. Curricula are expected to include philosophical approaches, outcomes, designs, courses, and evaluation strategies. Clinical practicums can be structured as courses in the curriculum, either as part of a theoretical course or as a stand-alone course. Clinical practicums must be considered in relation to available health-care facilities that are able to accommodate students.

Curricula in programs that educate future practitioners in health fields are strongly affected by requirements of professional associations, regulatory agencies, and approval boards (Melrose et al., 2020). Curricula must address discipline-specific competencies. Throughout the process of curricular planning, program planners from educational institutions must negotiate with administrators of service agencies to find suitable clinical practicum sites.

Since the education of health-care professionals now occurs in universities rather than in the agencies providing services, designing, negotiating, and evaluating clinical practicums in relation to the overarching curriculum is seldom a linear process. One consideration is *program structure* or the duration and division of learning to be undertaken by students. Here modes of delivery matter: program structure could be framed within face-to-face settings in traditional classrooms, distance delivery, or a blend of them. Partnerships between institutions and consortiums or collaborations among institutions also matter. When programs are structured to be delivered at a distance, learners might have to travel and find accommodations in different geographical areas in order to attend their practicums. In both face-to-face and distance programs, international practicum experiences might be available and even required.

Another consideration is the *program model* or organization of required courses, elective courses, laboratory experiences, and clinical practicums within the curriculum. In clinical practicums, the program model guides the method of instruction to be used. For example, the program model might require that students are taught in small groups by a clinical instructor, in one-to-one interaction with a preceptor, or in a combination of these and other instructional methods.

In the health disciplines, coordinating instruction extends well beyond the actual institutions of learning and into clinical agencies. Schedules, faculty appointments, and budgets must all be addressed. The instructors and preceptors who teach students during their clinical practicums might have no other association with the university. Similarly, university faculty assigned to teach in a particular clinical area might have no current association with a particular agency.

Program design configures the program of studies, including the courses selected, practicum experiences, relationships among courses, and policies that communicate this information. Designs can include building with blocks of required study, building by spiralling back and adding to previous content at different points, and establishing opportunities for specific tasks such as an essential psychomotor skill. Clinical teachers seldom have input into how programs are structured, the type of model used to organize content, or the design influencing how and when information is presented. However, all those involved in educating students must seek a basic understanding of the "big picture" curriculum that students follow.

Traditionally, curricular organizing strategies often revolved around the medical model. The hospital areas of medicine, surgery, pediatrics, maternity, and psychiatry framed the focus of learning for health practitioners. This model is strongly aligned with hospital-based apprenticeship orientations to learning and is now considered somewhat outdated in today's complex and ever-changing health-care system (Benner et al., 2010; Diekelmann, 2003; Tanner, 2006).

Today programs are more often organized within a conceptual framework generated in the discipline or around the outcomes expected of graduates. For example, with outcomes such as promoting health, thinking critically, and making decisions, curriculum planners would organize content related to each of these outcomes in different courses throughout the program. Methods of evaluation would be determined in relation to these outcomes, and they would include a wide range of educational measurements. Examples are multiple choice exams and scholarly papers in academic classes and skill mastery or client communication in clinical practicums.

Levelling is the process of linking program content, introduced at different times and in different courses, to the evaluated outcomes expected of graduates. Levelling requires planned opportunities for students to build on their previous knowledge and work incrementally toward achieving more complex outcomes. However, if a limited number of clinical placements are available, scheduling appropriate clinical opportunities for students at all levels is particularly challenging. Introductory-level students might find themselves in practicums in which they must care for acutely ill individuals. In many instances, practicum placements are more suited to advanced learners than to students in basic health-care programs.

Furthermore, instructors, staff members, and students can find it difficult to link the learning outcomes and evaluation methods that flow from a program's unique conceptual framework with the day-to-day work of a clinical agency. This might be another consequence of the limited associations between universities and clinical agencies. Although links between learning outcomes and day-to-day practice are made during planning by representatives of universities and agencies, the links might not always be clearly communicated to staff actually working with learners.

Admission criteria are another important curricular element in appreciating the complexities of planned aspects of clinical learning environments. Some learners come to a health-related program of study with less than a high school education. Others come to postsecondary education with high school completion but are introduced to a college, technical institute, or university for the first time. Still others have at least one level of certification or an undergraduate or graduate degree. At any level, qualifications for admission might have been completed in another country and in another language. Learners might also have been awarded credit for prior learning or transfer programs.

Clinical agencies often host learners from a variety of different programs, and admission requirements will be different for each program even within the same discipline. For example, whereas one registered nurse program might require high school completion, another might accept adult learners who have completed bridging programs. Inconsistent admission criteria among programs can leave agency staff members unsure of what learners are expected to know when they arrive, particularly when coupled with learning outcomes and evaluation methods that might not seem to be straightforward. In turn, staff can feel confused about how learners should be progressing and the specific task-based competencies that they should be achieving.

As a new clinical teacher, find out as much as possible about the overarching curriculum that directs your learners' program of study. What is the philosophical approach guiding the program? Go beyond considering expected student outcomes for the specific course that you are teaching and think deeply about the outcomes expected of students after they graduate. Visualize your present course in relation to the design of the program.

In the big picture, ask yourself how the course that you are teaching builds upon previous courses. Which specific skills or ways of thinking must students master to progress to the next level? Will supplemental activities be needed if opportunities to learn these foundational skills are not available? What are the methods being used to evaluate students in different courses? Are the methods of evaluation in the course that you are teaching familiar to students?

You can also consider the impact of admission criteria on the dynamics of your student group. For example, which life event factors might be distracting students from learning in the clinical environment? Could students away from home for the first time feel heightened anxiety? Could an adult learner who reverts to a student role feel hampered in self-confidence? Although none of these questions is likely to have an immediate or easy answer, sorting through the planned aspects of a program and their implications establishes a foundation for managing the less predictable and unexpected aspects.

Curricular structure, model, design, outcomes, evaluation methods, and admission requirements of a program are planned with great care. They offer big picture direction and open doors for learning in the clinical environment. Even so, unpredictable events are sure to emerge once clinical practicums are under way. In the following section, we discuss the heart of any clinical learning environment for many students, instructors, and staff, the unplanned aspects of clinical learning.

UNPLANNED EXPERIENCES

The clinical learning environment is equivalent to a classroom for students during their practicums (Chan, 2004), yet few clinical agencies resemble traditional classrooms. In their clinical classrooms, learners hope to integrate into agency routines and feel a sense of *belonging* (Levett-Jones et al., 2008). Learners want to feel welcome and accepted by staff, and they want staff to help teach them how to practise confidently and competently (Courtney-Pratt et al., 2011; Henderson et al., 2012). Students require and expect feedback on their performance, and they must have opportunities for non-evaluated student-teacher discussion time (Melrose & Shapiro, 1999) and critical reflection (Duffy, 2009; Forneris & Peden-McAlpine, 2009; Mohide & Matthew-Maich, 2007). Learners need time to progress from one level of proficiency to another (Benner, 2001). Just as learners in classroom environments need support to develop competence in their chosen professions, learners in clinical practicums need a supportive clinical learning environment.

Although supportive clinical classrooms are hoped for, clinical teachers must also be well prepared for unplanned experiences that raise barriers to learning. Research suggests that clinical learning environments might not be as supportive as learners would like. For example, Brown et al.'s (2011) work with undergraduate students from 10 different health disciplines reveals significant differences between learners' descriptions of their ideal learning environments and what they experience during their actual clinical practicums. Although participants in Brown et al.'s study express satisfaction with their learning experiences, they describe a mismatch between what they hoped for and what actually occurred. Similarly, recently graduated nurses indicate significant differences between the kinds of practicums that they deem good preparation for practice and those that they actually attended (Hickey, 2010).

Investigations of the experiences of physical therapy students were unable to define conclusively a *quality* learning environment, in part because of the diverse instructional practices by different community agencies overseeing students' practicums (McCallum et al., 2013). Over the past decade and in several different countries, student nurses rated their clinical experiences higher for their sense of achieving tasks but much lower for accommodating individual needs and views (Henderson et al., 2012).

Although university students are encouraged to question existing practice and the status quo, they find that staff in their clinical placements are seldom open to innovation or challenges to routine practices (Henderson et al., 2012).

Staff shortages, and other issues with which clinical agencies struggle, can leave students feeling that they are not receiving the direction that they need and that they are a burden to staff (Robinson et al., 2007). Students might feel alienation rather than the sense of belonging that they hope for (Levett-Jones et al., 2009). Students might express fear and discomfort in their relationships with staff (Cederbaum & Klusaritz, 2009, p. 423). Clinical learners have felt rejected, ignored, devalued, and invisible (Curtis et al., 2007). These findings suggest that in some instances health-care students are not receiving the support that they need.

By acknowledging that both unplanned and planned aspects of learning will occur in all clinical learning environments, educators can plan fitting responses. Clinical agencies will always have a professional duty to prioritize safe patient care over providing learners with clinical classrooms that align with their curricular and individual needs. As a consequence, and in spite of careful planning by university and agency program representatives, students might perceive their learning environment as unsupportive.

However, international leaders in the health disciplines are calling on clinical agency staff to view clinical teaching as part of their own professional development. They ask clinical agency staff to aid the next generation of professionals by striving to provide quality clinical learning environments in which students do feel supported (Courtney-Pratt et al., 2011; Koontz et al., 2010). Programs are testing new models of instruction (Franklin, 2010). Individual clinical teachers are striving to implement innovative teaching approaches that can create mutually beneficial connections between learners and staff during clinical practicums. Recognizing when unplanned aspects of clinical learning environments distract from students' learning is an important first step in triggering change. Evaluation surveys are one way to cast a spotlight on troublesome areas.

A Strategy to Try ▶ Giving Back

Knowing that students want to feel a sense of belonging in clinical agency staff groups, you can find ways for students to contribute. Encourage them to reach out to staff members with offers of help, no matter which tasks are involved. To establish a more reciprocal climate of knowledge exchange, reverse the one-way flow of information from staff to student. Share students' academic work with staff. For example, you can arrange students' input into existing in-service presentations or initiate new presentations. Whenever possible, record any presentations and make them available online so that those unable to attend can also benefit. Invite students to share relevant assignments from their courses that staff might value. Request space on agency bulletin boards (physical or electronic) and post these assignments. Help students to change the topics of posted assignments frequently, and keep the information shared as concise as possible.

Clinical Learning Environment Inventory. Surveys to measure the quality of clinical learning environments are available. For example, the Clinical Learning Environment Inventory (CLEI) was developed in Australia by Chan (2001, 2002, 2003) to measure student nurses' perceptions of psychosocial elements in clinical practicums. The CLEI consists of an "Actual" form that assesses the actual learning environment and a "Preferred" form that assesses what the student would like ideally in a learning environment. The CLEI is a self-report instrument with 42 items classified into six scales: personalization, student involvement, task orientation, innovation, satisfaction, and individualization. Students respond using a four-point Likert scale with the response options "Strongly agree," "Agree," "Disagree," and "Strongly disagree." Inventory factors of the instrument have been modified to include student centredness (Newton et al., 2010).

The CLEI has also been abbreviated to a 19-item scale measuring students' satisfaction with their actual learning environment in two aspects of their clinical experience: clinical facilitator support of learning and clinical learning environment. The Clinical Learning Environment Inventory-19 (CLEI-19; Salamonson et al., 2011) is shown in Table 2. The CLEI-19 can be used in formal processes of evaluation implemented by university program evaluators. It can also be used more informally by agency staff and clinical teachers interested in strengthening their clinical classroom environments.

Table 2—Abbreviated Clinical Learning Environment Inventory (CLEI-19)

SA = *Strongly agree*   A = *Agree*   D = *Disagree*   SD = *Strongly disagree*

1	The clinical facilitator was considerate of my feelings.	SA A D SD
2	The clinical facilitator talked to, rather than listened to me.	SA A D SD
3	I enjoyed going to my clinical placement.	SA A D SD
4	The clinical facilitator talked individually with me.	SA A D SD
5	I was dissatisfied with my clinical experiences on the ward/facility.	SA A D SD
6	The clinical facilitator went out of their way to help me.	SA A D SD
7	After the shift, I had a sense of satisfaction.	SA A D SD
8	The clinical facilitator often got sidetracked instead of sticking to the point.	SA A D SD
9	The clinical facilitator thought up innovative activities for students.	SA A D SD
10	The clinical facilitator helped me if I was having trouble with the work.	SA A D SD
11	This clinical placement was a waste of time.	SA A D SD
12	The clinical facilitator seldom got around to the ward/facility to talk to me.	SA A D SD
13	This clinical placement was boring.	SA A D SD
14	The clinical facilitator was not interested in the issues that I raised.	SA A D SD
15	I enjoyed coming to this ward/facility.	SA A D SD
16	The clinical facilitator often thought of interesting activities.	SA A D SD
17	The clinical facilitator was unfriendly and inconsiderate toward me.	SA A D SD
18	The clinical facilitator dominated debriefing sessions.	SA A D SD
19	This clinical placement was interesting.	SA A D SD

Note. Clinical facilitator support of learning component: Items 1, 2R, 4, 6, 8R, 9, 10, 12R, 14R, 16, 17R, 18R. Satisfaction with clinical placement: Items 3, 5R, 7, 11R, 13R, 15, 19. Items are scored 5, 4, 2, or 1 respectively for responses SA, A, D, and SD. Items marked with R are scored in the reverse manner. Omitted or invalidly answered items are scored 3. Adapted with permission (Salamonson et al., 2011).

Incidental learning. Adult educators Marsick and Watkins (1990, 2001) name learning that occurs as a by-product of doing something else incidental learning. Incidental or unintentional learning differs from formal learning, in which learners register with educational institutions to complete a program of study. Incidental learning also differs from informal learning, in which learners intentionally seek further information, for example, by joining a study group.

Although incidental learning is unplanned, learners are aware after the experience that learning has occurred. Incidental learning occurs frequently while a person is completing a seemingly unrelated task, particularly in the workplace. It is situated, contextual, and social. It can happen when watching or interacting with others, from making mistakes, or from being forced to accept or adapt to situations (Kerka, 2000). Clinical practicums, both those that students find supportive and those that they do not find supportive, offer unprecedented opportunities for incidental learning. Tapping into these opportunities can turn potentially negative experiences into positive ones.

Opportunities to achieve required learning outcomes in a clinical course can seem to be elusive. Possibilities emerge for thinking outside the box when clinical teachers nurture relationships with agency staff members, both in their own and in other health-care disciplines. You can ask whether a student can shadow a practitioner from another discipline and then lead peers in a discussion on how elements of critical thinking are both the same and different across professions. When appropriate, consider pairing a student with a paraprofessional or non-professional staff member to strengthen specific psychomotor skills or an understanding of the contributions of others to care.

In sum, the clinical learning environment is one of the most important classrooms for pre-service students. This environment offers a range of planned and unplanned opportunities for learners to practise and achieve the competencies that they need. Clinical placements are in short supply for most disciplines and might not always be as supportive as learners hope. Clinical teachers can find foundational guidance for their own courses in curricular structure, model, design, outcomes, evaluation methods, admission requirements, and tactics for levelling student learning.

Both unplanned and planned aspects of learning must be expected. University training programs for health professionals are separate from most clinical agencies, so clinical staff responsible for guiding learners might not be fully aware of their programs. Instruments such as the CLEI -19 can serve as a measure of how students perceive their clinical practicums. Ensuring that incidental or accidental learning is acknowledged and celebrated can begin to turn potentially negative clinical experiences into times of valuable learning.

WHO ARE THE TEACHERS?

Teaching in the health-care professions is a dynamic process. Practitioners can share their clinical expertise with novices beginning their careers or with more expert colleagues advancing their knowledge. One of the strongest motivators for becoming a clinical instructor is a desire to influence students' success and shape the next generation of health-care professionals in your discipline, ultimately influencing the quality of care provided by future practitioners (Penn et al., 2008). Clinical teachers are influential role models who continuously demonstrate professional skills, knowledge, and attitudes (Davies, 1993; Hayajneh, 2011; Janssen et al., 2008; Mohammadi et al., 2020; Okoronkwo et al., 2013; Perry, 2009).

BECOMING A CLINICAL TEACHER

The influence of employment category. Employment categories exert an important influence on the clinical teaching role. Some clinical teachers are full- or part-time employees of universities or agencies hosting clinical practicums. Workloads for these teachers are negotiated with their employers, and they are given release time for preparation and attendance in their assigned clinical areas. Other clinical teachers might be employed only on a contract basis.

Over the past decade, contract faculty have become the new majority at universities (Charfauros & Tierney, 1999; Gappa, 2008; Meixner et al., 2010). Contracts can offer positions such as limited-term full-time faculty (Rajagopal, 2004), part-time faculty, sessional instructors, term instructors (Puplampu, 2004), and adjunct faculty (Meixner et al., 2010). These faculty "are paid per course taught and are seldom offered benefits such as health insurance or access to retirement plans" (Meixner et al., 2010, p. 141). Clinical teachers can be employed in different ways and at several different institutions.

Although contract employment offers employees flexibility and independence, workers who are employed on a contract basis might feel less secure in their jobs, and their sense of well-being can be negatively affected (Bernhard-Oettel et al., 2008). Contract employees can feel marginalized and disadvantaged (Guest, 2004).

In university health-care programs, PhD qualifications are usually required for permanent academic positions, leaving many highly skilled practitioners underqualified (Jackson et al., 2011). Often clinical teachers continue their own education through graduate studies at the master's or doctoral level while they are instructing in clinical practicums. However, contract work might not accommodate the time that clinical teachers need to complete assignments for their own studies or to attend to family matters. Given the high demand for placements at clinical agencies, the times that students are scheduled to attend practicums cannot be altered, and substitute instruction is seldom available.

Uncertainty about whether their limited employment contracts will be continued can leave clinical teachers hesitant to risk implementing new ideas. Students' evaluations of teachers can reflect issues that are beyond teachers' control, yet these evaluations influence contract renewals. Student feedback is the main form of assessment of clinical teachers (Center for Research on Teaching and Learning, 2014; Fong & McCauley, 1993; Kelly, 2007). For some practitioners, contract employment with a university can seem to be less predictable than a clinical agency position.

A Strategy to Try ▶ *What Happens When I'm Ill?*

When a clinical teacher is ill, which steps are in place to arrange for a substitute teacher? When substitute teachers are unavailable, which additional steps are in place to notify the clinical agency and all members of the student group that the clinical experience will be cancelled?

If no formal steps are outlined at the curricular level, then establish a plan with your group of students. For example, draft a phone list in which each student is responsible for notifying the student whose name is next on the list. Each student must contact the designated peer until the last student reports to the first that the fan-out is complete. Keeping this list up to date will save students the inconvenience of arriving at their clinical placement only to find that they are unable to work because their clinical teacher is ill. For some students, privacy issues might be a concern, and opt-outs must always be available.

In most instances, becoming a clinical teacher involves self-orientation to the practicum placement area. Instructors who are new to the particular clinical setting in which they will be teaching or who have not practised there recently often choose to "buddy" or partner with an experienced staff member. Teresa Evans shares the following suggestions.

1. Call and make an appointment for your buddy shifts (it is often good to do 2 days in a row).
2. Make an appointment to meet with the unit manager during that time. It is good to know that everyone is starting on the same page, and clear communication from the beginning is essential. Some things to discuss with the unit manager include the following.
    a. Determine when you will start, how long you will be there, and which days of the week you will be there (roughly). The placement coordinator will send out a letter containing the relevant information to the facility in advance of your clinical starting date.
    b. Give the unit manager a course outline and talk a bit about what you hope students will get out of this clinical experience.
    c. Briefly go over the assignments that the students are to do during the course.
    d. Ask the unit manager about their expectations of you and the students. (What worked well in the past? What would the manager like to change?)
    e. Discuss your expectations of the staff.
3. Go through policies and procedures that will be used during the course of the clinical experience (e.g., administering blood and blood products).
4. Ask the staff which typical skills, conditions, and interventions they see or perform on a regular basis. Ask questions about them. You might want to find some research on them for your clinical binder.
5. Understand how the normal routine of the day goes.
    a. When are meals?
    b. When are vital signs typically taken if they are routine?
    c. How often is bedding changed? Where does soiled linen go?
    d. Get help learning how to use the assist tub if necessary.
    e. Where is report taken? When does report occur?
    f. What are the physio/occupational therapy schedules?

6. Look through the charts and have someone run through typical charting for the day and expectations regarding times of completion.
7. Do an admission or have someone walk you through the admission process.
8. What needs to be done for discharges? Transfers?
9. Orientate yourself to where all the supplies are. Go through all storage areas so that you know where everything is.
10. How are medications given and by whom? Do students usually have a separate binder for their own patients? Who has keys to the medication carts, and how many are there?
11. Your primary role during your buddy shift is to get to know the staff and have them get to know you. Also discuss what you and the students will be doing on the floor.
    a. Clarify which year the students are in.
    b. Mention which skills they can do (it can be helpful to bring a year skills list and post it for the staff).
    c. Determine the role that you need the staff to fulfill.
    d. Clarify what the students will do on the floor (e.g., charting, vital signs, bed baths, etc.).
    e. State your expectations of the staff.
12. Do morning care, assessments, and vital signs, and then ask to chart and have a staff member look over the information to make sure that it is complete.
13. Talk with the unit clerk, the crucial gatekeeper of information. Ask the clerk what typically happens when orders are received, where to put charts, how orders are processed, what to do if supplies need to be ordered, and so on. Unit clerks sometimes have concerns about students, especially when they take charts and do not understand orders that need to be processed, so discuss this with them in advance.
14. Look through patient charts to get a feel for how they are set up and what types of patients the unit generally receives.
15. Are there clipboards on which vital signs are recorded? Where are they recorded in the charts?
16. Ask staff how they know if samples (urine, sputum, etc.) need to be collected?

17. Ask about which certifications are needed to work on the floor. It might be prudent to talk to the appropriate individual and see if you can set up a date and time to complete these certifications if necessary (e.g., IV starts and central lines).

18. Are there teaching tools that the unit uses for patients? Review them so that you are familiar enough with them to alert students to them when they need them.

19. If you are not familiar with any of the equipment, then arrange an in-service (e.g., IV pumps, vital machines, glucometers, lifts, etc.).

Hint: Instructors set an example for students to follow. Ensure you are as prepared as possible.

Nursing is a team profession. Encourage your students to embrace interdisciplinary team work where appropriate.

TERESA EVANS, MN, NURSING INSTRUCTOR, GRANDE PRAIRIE REGIONAL COLLEGE

Transitioning from practitioner to educator. As with any career change, the transition from practitioner to educator can cause feelings of anxiety, isolation, and uncertainty (Anderson, 2008; Dempsey, 2007; Heathcote & Green, 2021; Jetha et al., 2016; Little & Milliken, 2007; McDermid et al., 2013; Penn et al., 2008; Rodger, 2019). Although specific tasks required of clinical teachers can be learned, the language, culture, and practices of a university can be unfamiliar and difficult to grasp (Penn et al., 2008). For many practitioners, discussing specific expectations of the faculty role both formally with program leaders and informally with other teachers can help.

Competencies expected of clinical teachers (Robinson, 2009) include

- being both a skilled practitioner and a skilled educator;
- having excellent interpersonal and professional communication skills;
- implementing a range of assessment and evaluation methods;
- possessing leadership and administrative skills; and
- maintaining professional development and scholarship activities.

Juggling the roles of practitioner and educator and feeling as though they must be near perfect in both, can leave clinical teachers feeling threatened (Griscti et al., 2005). The professional development activities required to gain and retain competence in each role are different. Practitioners must continue to provide client care in new and different ways and attend in-service workshops on new skills, products, and equipment being used in their clinical agencies. Educators must integrate knowledge from the discipline of education, understand student-centred approaches to learning, and initiate a scholarly program of research and publication. Common to both roles are keeping up to date with research findings, attending conferences or other educational events, and undertaking self-directed study projects.

Moving beyond simply maintaining competence and toward excellence in the two roles takes time. At different points in their careers, clinical teachers might commit more time and effort to one role than the other. New clinical teachers who are experienced practitioners might focus initially on understanding the educator competency of assessing and evaluating learners.

Once novice clinical teachers gain expertise and confidence as university faculty members, they can collaborate with experienced researchers and authors to complete scholarly activities. At other times, clinical teachers might find it helpful to return to practice and strengthen their clinical expertise. Mentorship from more experienced faculty can help clinical teachers to establish and work toward achieving realistic career goals (Billings & Kowalski, 2008).

A Strategy to Try ▶ *Plan to Advance Your Career*

Review your employment category in relation to your long-term career goals. Whether your employment is contract based and renewable on a per course basis or a continuing part-time or full-time position, evaluate how it fits with your plans for advancement. Question the specific impact of student feedback on your performance or your employment status.

How can you arrange opportunities for professional development? Which processes are in place for discussing your career trajectory with your employer(s)? Are any leave or release time packages available for completing further graduate study?

Investigate options that might be available for continuing your professional education. Consider both online and face-to-face programs. During any graduate course of study, be sure to plan several hours of study time most days, particularly when assignments are due.

Practice can help to ease the transition from practitioner to educator. Facilitating engaging post-conferences is a skill that many new clinical teachers in the health professions must learn. Yet how does one learn to facilitate a clinical post-conference? Is it possible to learn this from trial and error? Does it help to discuss the role during a clinical instructor orientation session? Might it be helpful to be mentored and watch an experienced teacher facilitate a post-conference?

These are questions that Mary Ann Fegan at the University of Toronto thought about as she prepared new and returning instructors to facilitate clinical post-conferences. Many identified this aspect of their role to be challenging, and they wondered how to do the role better. Some asked, "How do I ensure that every student has a voice and feels comfortable participating in the discussion?"

Mary Ann and her colleague used the following active learning strategy to help prepare instructors for their facilitator role during clinical post-conferences. They find it to be an effective and fun way to address some of the challenges of the role and a great way to facilitate active discussion among both new and returning instructors. This activity uses role playing to simulate a post-conference.

Participants (instructors) are divided into small groups of six or seven people. One person volunteers to be the facilitator, and everyone else is handed a nursing student "role card." The role card provides a brief description of the student, and participants are invited to take on that role as they think it would play out in a real situation. Among the student roles are the following: a quiet student who only speaks when spoken to; a bored or unengaged student; a very chatty student who has an answer or comment for almost everything; an English language learner student who provides very short answers to questions; a dominant student who has had a great clinical day and wants to talk about everything that she or he did; and an anxious student who arrives a few minutes late and is very distraught about something that happened earlier that day. The simulation typically runs for about 15–20 minutes.

This activity is followed by small group debriefing (about 20 minutes) led by a faculty member who observed the small group discussion and took some notes. As with any simulated activity, the debriefing opens with a general question to help the group decompress, something like "How did that feel?" The discussions are rich and provide some interesting and insightful perspectives and observations from participants. Many questions are raised, and many are answered, among both new and returning instructors. This opportunity for peer-to-peer feedback helps to reveal some of the challenges in facilitating a group and offers some specific strategies to enhance this role. After the small group debriefings, everyone comes together for a larger group discussion and shares some of the things that went well, some that could have been done differently (in the spirit of wondering), and finally one key learning about the facilitator role.

MARY ANN FEGAN, MN, SENIOR LECTURER, CLINICAL EDUCATION COORDINATOR, LAWRENCE S. BLOOMBERG FACULTY OF NURSING, UNIVERSITY OF TORONTO

EFFECTIVE CLINICAL TEACHERS

The identity of clinical teachers as individuals, practitioners, and educators has a significant impact on their effectiveness in the clinical learning environment. How instructors understand the process of learning will ultimately guide how they go about teaching (Hand, 2006). Rather than simply teaching as they were taught, clinical teachers are now actively seeking ways to strengthen the scholarship of educating learners in clinical learning environments (Buccieri et al., 2013; Sabog et al., 2015; Schmutz et al., 2013).

If we view the clinical environment through the eyes of students, then it is not unexpected that learners perceive effective teachers as individuals who demonstrate caring behaviours (Jahangiri et al., 2013), who have high emotional intelligence (Mosca, 2019), who are calm during stressful experiences (Smith et al., 2011), who exercise patience (Cook, 2005; Parsh, 2010), and who demonstrate enthusiasm for their profession and for teaching (Gaberson & Oermann, 2010). Teachers who are approachable can help students to feel less anxious and more confident (Chitsabesan et al., 2006; Sieh & Bell, 1994). Students appreciate teachers who make themselves available outside of clinical time, who take the time to answer questions without seeming to be annoyed, and who provide students with time to debrief and discuss issues (Berg & Lindseth, 2004). Students find it helpful when teachers are not controlling or overly cautious and allow students to learn the practice skills that they need by actually doing them (Masunaga &

Hitchcock, 2011). In short, students value respectful collegial relationships with their teachers (Kelly, 2007).

Effective and student-centred clinical teachers empower their students. Empowering teaching behaviours include enhancing students' confidence, involving students in making decisions and setting goals, making learning meaningful for them, and helping them to become more autonomous professionals in their discipline (Babenko-Mould et al., 2012). Empowering teachers care about, commit to, and create with their students toward a shared vision that anything is possible (Chally, 1992).

Empowering strategies that foster a shared vision between clinical teachers and students include inviting students to identify the kinds of approaches that best support their learning styles (Melrose, 2004). Effective teachers support students in identifying their personal strengths and working with their teachers to build on these strengths (Cederbaum & Klusaritz, 2009). Empowering educators affirm students' efforts, share positive messages, and create supportive dynamics within the learning group (Chally, 1992). Note that empowering strategies also redirect students when their work is unsatisfactory or off track.

In higher education settings, educators must assess and evaluate students' work, thus affording educators power over whether students can continue in a course or program. The inherent tension in holding power over students while seeking to empower them or share power with them is not easily resolved. Ultimately, clinical teachers must determine students' grades, whether students are capable of practising safely in their discipline, and whether students can progress in their chosen field.

A Strategy to Try ▶ *Remember a Favourite Teacher*

Consider your own learning experiences and reflect on teachers whom you have known. Does a favourite teacher come to mind? Recall the characteristics of this teacher as an individual who stands out in your memory in both positive and negative ways. How does this individual, and other teachers whom you have known, influence your teaching? Who are the role model teachers whom you would like to emulate?

Think about writing down these reflections. With the positive memories, would it be fitting to email or send a letter to the special teacher who came to mind?

A Strategy to Try ▶ *Do a Reflection Inventory*

Imagine doing a reflection inventory of your own teaching. How might students describe you as a teacher? Would their descriptions include words such as *calm, patient, enthusiastic,* and *approachable*? Would they view you as available and willing to take time to answer questions or debrief with them? Would they describe you as the professional whom they aspire to be?

A Strategy to Try ▶ *Find Education-Focused Journals and Conferences*

Which elements of your teaching practice are "teaching as you were taught"? In contrast, which elements of your teaching practice implement an idea gleaned from a journal article or a conference presentation grounded in the discipline of education? Find an education-focused journal in your discipline and make a point of reading articles regularly. Attend professional conferences focused on teaching and learning.

A Strategy to Try ▶ *Anything Is Possible*

Consider the concept of empowering learners. Working from the premise that anything is possible, invite students to articulate what they hope to achieve during their learning and how they will go about achieving it. Find ways to build on their own ways of learning.

A Strategy to Try ▶ *Balance Affirmations and Corrections*

Tune in to the number of affirmations that you express in your discussions with students. Are messages of correction, redirection, and even failure balanced with messages of support and positive regard?

Once you identify the learning needs of students in clinical settings, you might have difficulty knowing the best strategy to support their learning and provide the safest care to patients. To address students' and clinical instructors' learning needs for clinical issues, instructors at Lakehead University conduct a general orientation at the beginning of each clinical session.

Clinical instructors from all year levels are asked to attend. The instructors range from those who have many years of experience in the clinical area to those who are just starting. We begin the session by asking the experienced instructors to describe how they orient students to the clinical area. This usually stimulates questions from the new instructors.

We then ask the instructors to give examples of challenges that they have faced in the clinical area. This again stimulates questions about formal documentation and how the clinical instructor can seek guidance from faculty and other instructors.

Feedback from the clinical instructors has been very positive. They get a chance to hear what the challenges are in each year level, to know who else is teaching in the program, and to learn who can contribute to the conversation with their own experiences. The instructors have developed a greater sense of connection. We would like to make this an even more inter-active experience by having the clinical instructors role-play a situation in a clinical setting and then have feedback from the entire group.

CATHY SCHOALES, MN, FACULTY OF NURSING, LAKEHEAD UNIVERSITY

In sum, clinical teachers are role models who serve their profession by nurturing and supporting the next generation of practitioners. Clinical teachers affiliated with university programs can be employed in different ways. They can be part-time or full-time continuing faculty, or they can be employed on time-limited contracts for each course taught. They can work for several different learning institutions and clinical agencies. Given that finding substitutes to cover clinical teaching commitments is difficult, instructors should establish contingency plans such as student phone lists for when they are ill.

In most instances, full-time faculty are qualified at the PhD level. Often clinical teachers undertake graduate studies at the same time as they instruct in clinical practicums. Planning time to complete your own study assignments while teaching is essential.

The process of transitioning from practitioner to educator can seem to be overwhelming. Expectations of university faculty members might not always be clear. Seeking mentors and collaborating with experienced faculty involved in research and publication activities can help new clinical teachers to develop their own programs of scholarship. As both educators and practitioners, clinical teachers must gain and maintain competence in both areas. At different times in their careers, clinical teachers might focus more on one set of these competencies.

In addition to demonstrating competence and expertise in their discipline, effective clinical teachers project a calm, patient, approachable, and enthusiastic attitude during their interactions with students. Effective clinical teachers go beyond what is required of them and find ways to empower and inspire students with the idea that anything is possible. Whether students are progressing well, need redirecting, or are failing, effective clinical teachers work from a student-centred approach based on student strengths to affirm and support students.

WHO ARE THE STUDENTS?

Like snowflakes, no two students are alike. Learners who come to clinical areas of health care can be young adults beginning their higher education at a local college or university, they can be adult learners just launching their university learning, or they might have already completed undergraduate or graduate degrees. Students might be living at home with their families or far away in new locations. Some might have been awarded advanced credits. Others might have been educated in different countries and have cultural orientations that are unfamiliar to teachers, peers, or agency staff. In addition to their studies, many university students are employed either part time or full time. Many students have extensive family responsibilities.

Despite this student diversity, teachers can expect that students in the health-care professions will find the clinical learning environment stressful, at least initially. Although all learners will experience and project emotions in unique ways, research suggests that commonalities exist. Students are likely to fear that they will harm patients, they want to help people, they need to integrate theory and clinical practice, and they desire to master psychomotor skills (O'Connor, 2006). Mastering those skills can seem to dominate what students view as most important during clinical practicums. After graduating, however, learners report that having time and opportunity to practise their communication, time management, and organizational skills is actually more important (Hartigan-Rogers et al., 2007).

The high cost of tuition is a concern for most university students. Coupled with living costs that can include travel to and additional accommodation at out-of-town clinical practicum sites, students face significant debt loads. Given the sacrifices that students make to earn credentials in their chosen health-care professions, understandably they usually expect to be awarded top marks and feel devastated when their efforts are graded as poor or failing.

A Strategy to Try ▶ *Value Students' Sacrifices*
What sacrifices have students in your group made to attend their educational program? What sacrifices have they made to attend the clinical placement? How can this information help you to understand your students?

A Strategy to Try ▶ *Arrange Practice Time*
Knowing that most students feel anxious at the beginning of their clinical placement, have them work closely with agency staff until their confidence increases. Arrange practice time to help students achieve competence with psychomotor skills whenever possible. Some agencies have resources such as simulation equipment with which learners can practise skills (discussed in more detail in Chapter 5). The clinical educator in the agency often has access to resources for orienting new staff.

A Strategy to Try ▶ *Organize Peer Support Opportunities*
Create opportunities for students to discuss their fears and their coping strategies to resolve those fears. Provide activities for students to work with partners or small groups. Peer support can be invaluable.

Students, teachers, clinical agency staff, and patients come from different backgrounds and have different perspectives and ways of interacting. These diverse perspectives become apparent in clinical practicums as students are required to communicate with individuals with whom they have little in common. One way of understanding these perspectives is to consider learners, teachers, patients/clients, and health-care team members with whom they must interact in relation to cultural, intergenerational, and emotional diversity.

CULTURAL DIVERSITY

The term "culture," which broadly refers to people's way of life, can have many meanings. The term includes the standards, morals, principles, and experiences that influence how people think and behave (Sonn & Vermeulen, 2018). Age, gender, ethnicity, race, language, religion, spiritual tradition, and sexual orientation all contribute to the diverse cultural identities that individuals and groups affiliate with or are influenced by (Garneau & Pepin, 2015; Melrose et al., 2020). Each affiliation can influence what people value, how they express themselves, and how they carry out their activities of daily living.

Although health professionals are expected to demonstrate knowledge and understanding of and sensitivity to the expressions of cultural diversity that they encounter when caring for patients or clients, some people still receive unequal treatment (Jongen et al., 2018; Smedley et al., 2003). Similarly, in educational settings, some students in the health professions continue unfairly to receive unequal treatment (Guerra & Kurtz, 2016; Kruse et al., 2018; Smith, 2018).

Cultural competence requires health professionals to ensure that, at both individual and systemic levels, the agencies where they practise demonstrate "a set of congruent behaviours, attitudes, and policies that come together [to] . . . enable [people] . . . to work effectively in cross-cultural situations" (Cross et al., p. 28). Cultural competence in health professions education requires teachers to "adapt teaching and learning techniques in a way that values, empowers, and accommodates . . . student diversity. Cultural competence begins with an assessment of the learner's needs and includes student interactions, curricula and policy development, in-class and online considerations, culturally competent policies and procedures, and . . . educators committed to lifelong learning" (Smith, 2018, p. 20). Achieving needed cultural competence is an ongoing process by which teachers learn with (and from) students, patients, clients, agency practitioners, and fellow faculty members.

Cultural safety extends the concept of cultural competence beyond efforts to understand the kinds of behaviours in which people from different cultures engage. Cultural safety directly acknowledges that patients/clients or students receive unequal treatment and learning opportunities because an inherent power imbalance exists between them and their health-care providers or teachers. "This concept rejects the notion that health providers should focus on learning cultural customs of different ethnic groups. Instead, cultural safety seeks to achieve better care through being aware of difference, decolonising, considering power relationships, implementing reflective practice, and by allowing the patient [or student] to determine whether a clinical encounter is safe" (Curtis et al., 2019, p. 3).

Strengthening cultural competence and creating culturally safe learning environments for students centre on teachers becoming more self-aware through self-reflection. Acknowledging that teachers hold power and privilege in their relationships with their students is an important first step. Furthermore, Melrose et al. (2020) urged teachers to reflect deeply on their own cultures, beliefs, and imprinted stereotypes. In turn, when teachers question how their personal views affect their teaching, they are better equipped to help their students feel safe and to meet their needs, expectations, and rights respectfully. Ultimately, teachers who are committed to demonstrating cultural safety participate in practices that challenge stereotypes, structural racism, and systemic inequities in health care and in the education of health-care professionals.

A Strategy to Try ▶ *Cultural Competence Self-Reflection*

Consider the following questions as you reflect on how your own culture affects your teaching.

1. How do I share information about my age, gender, ethnicity, race, language, religion, spiritual tradition, and sexual orientation with other people? With my students?
2. Which stereotypical beliefs do I hold about people from cultures different from my own?

3. When has my own cultural perspective influenced my judgment about what "normal" or "appropriate" behaviours, values, and communication styles should look like in my students?
4. Which opportunities are available for me to incorporate cultural competence and cultural safety into my teaching practice?

INTERGENERATIONAL DIVERSITY

Although the term "diversity" is often used in relation to the cultural affiliations mentioned above, diversification can also occur when multiple generations work or study together (Fry, 2011; Johnson & Romanello, 2005; Weston, 2006). Each generation grows up with different life experiences, which influence how members of a generational cohort view the world, how they communicate, and how they approach teaching and learning (Billings, 2004; Notarianni et al., 2009).

A generation is a group of people or cohort who progresses through time together, holding or sharing a common place in history. Each group shares social and political events that usually span from 15 to 20 years. As a result, members of that group view the world in a way different from generations born before and after them. However, we must not make assumptions that all individuals of a particular age will demonstrate characteristics associated with their cohort. In some instances, though, linking an individual's way of being in the world with characteristics expected of the generational group can be useful. Viewing learners and those with whom they interact through a generational lens can promote awareness of today's students, their expectations, and how teachers can respond to their needs (Earle & Myrick, 2009).

Currently, four active generations are interacting in schools, workplaces, homes, families, and communities (Gibson, 2009; Weston, 2006). These four generations are known as the Traditionalists or Veterans or Silent Generation, born between 1900 and 1945; Baby Boomers or Sandwich Generation, born between 1946 and 1964; Generation X or Nexers, born between 1965 and 1980; and Millennials or Generation Y or Net Generation, born between 1981 and 2002. A fifth generation, Generation Z, learners born after 1995, is now entering universities.

Students are most likely to meet Traditionalists as clients or patients during clinical practicums. Having lived through world wars and the Great Depression, those born during this period commonly experienced hardship. As a result, they worked hard, were loyal, and believed that the sacrifices they made would be rewarded (Tilka Miller, 2007). The world of this generation was very different from that of today. News came from newspapers and radios; shopping was done locally. Members of this generation were willing to conform to their parents' beliefs rather than rebel against them, and they have been able to adapt to changes in the world (Johnson & Romanello, 2005). Their early work environments had clearly defined hierarchies, with plainly outlined rules, roles, policies, and procedures that employees were required to implement (Weston, 2006).

In health-care environments, uniforms offered immediate explanations to this generation of who the health-care providers were and what could be expected of them. In today's fast-paced and technology-rich health-care environments, Traditionalists might be unsure of students' roles and find their explanations difficult to understand.

Baby Boomers, now in their 50s, 60s, and 70s, are the largest cohort working in health care (Fry, 2011). Students will meet members of this generation primarily as the clinical leaders and practitioners in their practicums. Many Boomers grew up in a healthy, flourishing economy in which hospitals and schools thrived. Positive social influences on this generation encouraged Baby Boomers to think as individuals from a young age, to express themselves creatively, and to speak out when not in agreement with others.

Many women of this generation were socialized into the primarily female professions of nursing or teaching since these educational opportunities were widely available (Hill, 2004). Women of the Boomer generation were the first to work outside the home. This resulted in appreciably different home lives for the next generations.

In response to growing up in an era of prosperity, Boomers were willing to work long hours to pursue their goals, often in a relentless manner that might have negatively affected their personal lives (Stewart & Torges, 2006). Boomers are now often sandwiched between caring for their aging parents and their adult children. They are also investing considerable time, effort, and money into health maintenance and retirement (Johnson & Romanello, 2005). Given their leadership roles and experiences in health care, Baby Boomers might be seen as intimidating by students.

Generation Xers, now in their 30s and 40s, are a much smaller group and have been referred to as a bridge between the generations born before and after the introduction of the internet (Wortsman & Crupi, 2009). They grew up with computers, video games, and microwaves, and they are comfortable and skilled using new technologies. They expect instant access to information.

Members of this cohort were raised by two working parents or by single mothers and thus became known as the "latchkey" generation. They learned to manage on their own, became resourceful, and increasingly relied on friends (Walker et al., 2006; Weston, 2006). Generation Xers have been described as having little regard for corporate life, are intent on challenging authority, and expect to have their opinions considered (Earle & Myrick, 2009; Walker et al., 2006; Weston, 2006).

In health-care environments, Generation Xers entered the workforce during the turbulent 1990s period of downsizing and restructuring. Many were unable to find full-time or continuous employment (Fry, 2011). As a result, they do not view employment as security (Hill, 2004). Opportunities for promotion can seem to be eclipsed by the Baby Boomers who remain in the workforce. Students will encounter Generation Xers among their peers, teachers, and clinical agency staff. Until relationships are forged, students can find Generation Xers to be impatient and somewhat unwilling to offer in-depth explanations.

Millennials, in their teens to their 30s, were raised by Boomers who were actively involved in their learning. They have high levels of self-confidence and close relationships with their parents and members of their parents' generation (Hill, 2004). Millennials are the second largest generational cohort in the general population (Buruss & Popkess, 2012; Wortsman & Crupi, 2009). They are fully comfortable with technology and with living in a diverse world. Millennials are considered the most culturally diverse generation of all time (Earle & Myrick, 2009; Walker et al., 2006).

This group of learners has a strong capacity to multitask, but their multitasking can erode their capacity to sustain focus and attention (Sherman, 2009). Their education has equipped them with the ability to work well collaboratively and on teams and to extend respect to each member of a group (Wortsman & Crupi, 2009). This cohort is accustomed to and requires immediate feedback (Bednarz, et al., 2010) and positive reinforcement (McCurry & Martins, 2010).

Millennials will be present in student, teaching, and staff groups. Students might find that individuals from this group are fun-loving, friendly, and approachable, particularly if students themselves are Millennials. Some members of this cohort might have had limited exposure to failure or even to negative feedback.

Generation Zers are people born after 1995 and comprise one-quarter of the North American population (Kingston, 2014). They lived through the terrorist bombings of 9/11 and the 2008 recession. Known as screenagers or digital natives, members of this cohort have grown up with the internet, social media, and smartphones, and they are considered the most connected generation in history (McCrindle & Wolfinger, 2014; Sparks & Honey, n.d.; Williams, 2019). Raised in inclusive classrooms, Generation Zers are collaborative, and over half will be university educated (Sparks & Honey, n.d.). They work quickly, can have short attention spans, communicate with symbols, and might not be precise or put effort into their writing (Sparks & Honey, n.d.). Assigned reading was identified as one of their least preferred methods of learning (Hampton, Welsh, & Wiggins, 2020).

Clinical teachers can use information about generational diversity as an introduction to who their students are and to create individualized instruction that will help them to succeed. The wisdom gleaned from Traditionalists, the drive modelled by Baby Boomers, the resourcefulness demonstrated by Generation Xers, the team spirit so ready to be tapped in Millennials, and the connectivity of Generation Zers can all be integrated into innovative teaching strategies.

A Strategy to Try ▶ *What's Your Generational Cohort?*
Question whether your students would benefit from viewing the individuals with whom they will be interacting professionally through the lens of generational diversity. During the process of coming to know your students, apply the strengths and weaknesses of their generational cohorts to enhance their learning outcomes.

Another way to understand the diverse perspectives that students bring to their clinical learning environment is to examine the diverse range of emotional issues that many face. Just as members of the general population deal with learning disabilities, substance abuse, poor mental health, or many other emotionally taxing problems, so too students who enrol in health-care programs deal with similar issues. Increased numbers of students with learning disabilities (Child & Langford, 2011; L'Ecuyer, 2019 a, 2019 b; McPheat, 2014; Meloy & Gambescia, 2014; Ridley, 2011; Sanderson-Mann et al., 2012), substance abuse problems (Monroe & Kenaga, 2010; Murphy-Parker, 2013), and poor mental health (Arieli, 2013; Megivern et al., 2003; Storrie et al., 2012) are successfully completing their programs. Although help and accommodation for these students are more readily available, the stigma associated with their issues makes students reluctant to share the challenges through which they are working.

Clinical teachers are not, and should not be, learning disability specialists or addiction and mental health counsellors. They must know, however, which program resources are available to students. All clinical teachers, whether they are full-time continuing faculty or teaching only one clinical course, should visit their university counselling centre and become fully informed about the services offered.

Most accommodations for learning disabilities are geared to academic class activities. For example, students with dyslexia benefit from supplemental study skills modules (Wray et al., 2013). If these kinds of modules are available, then clinical teachers should familiarize themselves with the content and highlight its clinical applicability during clinical conference discussions. Doing so would normalize the use of such resources. Non-dyslexic students might also find the supplemental activities a useful way to transfer theory to practice.

Research is beginning to reveal more about the nature of the difficulties experienced by learning disabled students in clinical placements. For example, dyslexic nursing students have more trouble writing notes about patients and using care plans than non-dyslexic students (Morris & Turnbull, 2006). Dyslexic students struggle with clinical documentation, drug calculations, and handovers of patients (Sanderson-Mann et al., 2012). They experience the most stress when the clinical environment is busy (Crouch, 2019).

Supports established in the academic setting might not be communicated to those instructing and precepting students in the clinical setting (Howlin et al., 2014). Staff nurses responsible for the clinical education of students and new nurses receive little preparation for that role and might not feel supported to meet the needs of those with learning difficulties (L'Ecuyer, 2019a). Preceptors can feel unprepared and lack confidence in their ability to instruct students who have learning disabilities (L'Ecuyer, 2019b).

Learning disabled students state that they would benefit from time spent with a clinical placement mentor who understands their specific learning issues (Child & Langford, 2011). Early referral and testing of students experiencing difficulties associated with dyslexia should be encouraged so that they can receive support as soon as possible (Ridley, 2011).

Focusing on abilities offers important balance in any discussion of disabilities. Individuals with learning disabilities have been characterized as focused, resilient, empathetic, compassionate, and intuitive, and they are known to have excellent interpersonal and problem-solving skills (Wray et al., 2013). These attributes are highly valued in health-care practitioners. Many clinicians with learning disabilities have found suitable strategies to overcome their learning difficulties and are thriving in their field.

The incidence of substance abuse among health-care professionals and students is both under-researched and under-reported, but from 10% to 15% of health-care professionals are estimated to be afflicted with alcohol or drug addiction (Monroe & Kenaga, 2010). In most jurisdictions, reporting is mandatory when any professional or student is impaired. When a clinical teacher encounters an impaired student, that student must be sent off the clinical area immediately, and the incident must be reported to the teacher's supervisor. With this action, safety must be considered in areas such as finding alternative transportation if the student drove to the clinical site. Instructor and student should agree to discuss the incident when the student is no longer impaired.

Neither students nor practitioners should ever practise when impaired. Unfortunately, individuals with substance abuse issues might not believe that they have a problem and thus be reluctant to seek help. When clinical teachers identify substance abuse or the potential for substance abuse in their students and initiate referrals to university counselling services, they provide a critical lifeline. Throughout the world, programs are becoming available that offer confidential, non-punitive assistance for health-care professionals and students suffering from addictions (Monroe & Kenaga, 2010). Ignoring issues related to substance abuse is not an option.

Students with emotional problems are also present across health-care disciplines and in clinical placements. Learners with mental health issues can demonstrate inappropriate behaviours, including anger, neediness, and inability to complete tasks (Storrie et al., 2012). They can display poor motivation, negativity, overconfidence, or inability to work as a member of the health-care team. They might not accept responsibility for their actions or change their behaviour in response to feedback.

In response, clinical teachers can feel anxious, distressed, intimidated, or unsure about what to do (Storrie et al., 2012). When students present with a psychiatric or mental health crisis, they must be accompanied to an emergency treatment facility. In non-emergency situations, the best course of action is less clear. University counselling services are not immediately available to students when they are in practice areas. Other members of the student group, as well as agency clients and staff, will be affected by any inappropriate student behaviour.

Storrie et al. (2012, p. 101) suggest the following four strategies that clinical teachers can consider when responding to students with poor mental health.

1. Communicate with colleagues in advance about high-risk students who might have special needs in a clinical placement.
2. Maintain a consistent approach by following university procedures. If students have a complaint, then they are to address it first at a local level with clinical teachers. If the complaint is not resolved, then students must formalize it via a letter to a university supervisor.
3. Keep a clear audit trail by documenting any encounter with the student and regularly briefing your immediate supervisor.
4. Determine if the problem can be managed by rearranging the design of the student's study plan. A revised plan will consider the student's needs and strengths but still maintain academic expectations.

A Strategy to Try ▶ *Know Policies for Dealing with Emotionally Diverse Students*
In your self-orientation to your clinical teaching practice, find out precisely
which actions are required of you when you encounter students with learning disabilities, substance abuse, or poor mental health. Obtain copies of
relevant policies.

A Strategy to Try ▶ *Meet Counselling and Learning Services Staff*
Walk into the counselling and learning services offices of the academic
institution to experience how students might feel when they seek help.
Make a point of meeting the resource staff members who are available to
students. Providing students with the names of resource staff when referring them can make the process more familiar and comfortable.

A Strategy to Try ▶ *Make a Wellness Plan*
Invite all students in your clinical teaching group to prepare personal
wellness plans. Encourage them to include physical and mental health
issues and strategies for coping. Provide an option for them to share their
wellness plans with you or an agency staff member with whom they will
be highly involved. Students troubled by emotional problems can find it
easier to disclose problems in writing, as part of a group activity, than in
one-to-one dialogue with a teacher who will be evaluating them.

From the Field ▶ *Keep a Pride Journal*

Throughout the course of a clinical day, have students note when they feel
good about something that they have done. Encourage them to experience
the feelings and then jot down the experiences. In the post-conference, have
them share those experiences and discuss how they felt proud of what they did.

Mary Ellen Bond (2009) has examined the detrimental effects that
negative emotions such as shame can have on students' ability to learn in
clinical nursing education. Keeping a pride journal introduces an opportunity for students to articulate and celebrate positive emotions, those times
when they felt proud.

MARY ELLEN BOND, RN, MSN, COLLEGE OF THE ROCKIES

DEVELOPING INDEPENDENCE

Health-care students can be culturally, generationally, or emotionally diverse, but they share the common goal of needing to develop professional independence during their clinical practicums. Through a stepwise process of gradually decreasing direction and guidance from teachers and agency staff, learners must work toward practising independently. University-educated professionals in health-care fields are required to think and act on their own, with limited or no direction from professional colleagues. A crisis is an everyday occurrence. Once learners graduate, they will be expected to implement client care independently.

The processes and strategies that learners use to develop independence as practitioners are inherently difficult to understand. Seminal literature from the field of adult education indicates that a key element of developing independence in any educational activity is for students to take responsibility for their learning above and beyond responding to instructions (Boud, 1988; Knowles, 1975). Becoming independent requires students to choose suitable learning activities, reflect on their effectiveness, and initiate any needed changes (Holec, 1981; Little, 1991).

In chaotic clinical learning environments, in which maintaining patient safety is critical, students can feel unsure about how they could or should go beyond what they have been instructed to do. There is an inherent tension between providing safe patient care and initiating new or perhaps unfamiliar activities in clinical practicums. Ameliorating that tension is different from trying new ideas in academic classroom settings. Students might not feel that they have developed the independence they need to function in a complex professional role until nearly a year after they graduate (Melrose & Wishart, 2013).

A Strategy to Try ▸ *Where Do You Hope to Practise?*
Ask your students to name the clinical areas in which they hope to practise after graduation. Throughout the clinical placement, link any learning experiences to the specific competencies that they will need in those areas. With the goal of developing student independence, intentionally decrease support over the term of the practicum. Students cannot be expected to practise independently in all areas of the clinical placement. Clinical teachers can help to increase students' confidence, however, by focusing on skills directly relevant to their intended practice areas.

In sum, students in the health-care professions are a diverse group. Some will be new to university, and others will be experienced adult learners. Despite differences in their backgrounds, they can all be expected to be highly invested in their education, and they will have made sacrifices to complete clinical practicums. Most will feel anxious initially, particularly in their desire to provide safe care to patients and to pass course requirements.

Student groups will include learners from different cultures. Clinical teachers can support and celebrate their diversity by intentionally developing cultural competence and striving to create culturally safe learning environments. They can best do so by acknowledging the power that they hold in teacher-student relationships and engaging in ongoing self-reflection on how their own beliefs influence their teaching.

The groups will also include students from different generations. Clinical teachers can find it helpful to come to know their students as members of a generational cohort. Students will meet Traditionalists or older adults as clients/patients and Baby Boomers or middle-aged adults as clinical leaders and practitioners. They will meet Generation Xers in their 30s and 40s and Millennials in their 20s and 30s in peer, instructor, and agency staff groups. They will meet Generation Zers in their 20s in peer groups. Traditionalists are known for their wisdom and experience, Baby Boomers for their leadership and drive, Generation Xers for their resourcefulness and willingness to challenge, Millennials for their confidence and team spirit, and Generation Zers for their ability to work collaboratively.

Student groups will also include learners with emotionally diverse needs related to learning disabilities, substance abuse, or poor mental health. To accommodate these learners and ensure public safety, clinical teachers must have a clear understanding of any program resources and policies relevant to students with special needs. Key strategies for supporting troubled students include documenting both students' behaviours and teachers' responses implemented to help and consistently keeping supervisors informed.

Students and teachers in clinical learning environments share the goal of developing independent practitioners. Becoming independent is work in progress for students, teachers, and clinicians alike. By grounding instruction in the premise that students will soon be on their own and responsible for their practice, the importance of supporting students toward initiating and managing their own learning becomes clear.

CONCLUSION

Clinical environments are "classrooms" rich with planned, unplanned, and incidental opportunities for creative teaching and meaningful learning. Some clinical placements might not be as supportive as learners would like, and clinical agency staff might not be fully aware of students' programs. Still, more practitioners are embracing the view that supporting students is a valuable part of their own professional development.

Clinical teachers, whether they are continuing faculty members or employed only on a course-by-course basis, are impactful role models who can make a critical difference in their students' lives. Students view effective clinical teachers as individuals who are calm, patient, enthusiastic, and approachable. Excellent teachers seek to empower and inspire their students. Clinical teachers are often continuing their own graduate studies and juggling career plans that require expertise in both their practice discipline and the field of education.

The students whom clinical teachers meet in clinical practicums come from diverse cultural and generational backgrounds. Some will need unique instructional and institutional support as they deal with issues such as learning disabilities, substance abuse, or poor mental health. Clinical teachers must familiarize themselves with policies related to students with special needs and with counselling resources that are available to students. The stakes are high in university health-care programs, and all students have made sacrifices. They want to succeed, to earn top marks, and to practise independently once they graduate.

In this chapter, we examined the clinical learning environment and clarified the teachers and students in that environment. We hope that the creative strategies mentioned will provide practical ideas to help clinical teachers with the complex problems that they face daily. Perhaps the process of questioning and seeking to understand how our learners see the clinical environment is as important as the answers themselves.

REFERENCES

Anderson, J. (2008). An academic fairy tale: A metaphor of the work-role transition from clinician to academician. *Nurse Educator, 33*(2), 79–82.

Arieli, D. (2013). Emotional work and diversity in clinical placements of nursing students. *Journal of Nursing Scholarship, 45*(2), 192–201. https://doi.org/10.1111/jnu.12020

Babenko-Mould, Y., Iwasiw, C., Andrusyszyn, M., Spence Laschinger, H., & Weston, W. (2012). Nursing students' perceptions of clinical teachers' use of empowering teaching behaviours: Instrument psychometrics and application. *International Journal of Nursing Education Scholarship, 9*(1), Art. 5. https://doi.org/10.1515/1548-923X.2245

Bednarz, H., Schim, S., & Doorenbos, A. (2010). Cultural diversity in nursing education: Perils, pitfalls, and pearls. *Journal of Nursing Education, 49*(5), 253–260.

Benner, p. (2001). *From novice to expert: Excellence and power in clinical nursing practice.* (Commemorative ed.). Pearson Education.

Benner, P., Sutphen, M., Leonard, V., & Day, L. (2010). *Educating nurses: A call for transformation.* Jossey-Bass.

Berg, C., & Lindseth, G. (2004). Students' perspectives of effective and ineffective nursing instructors. *Journal of Nursing Education, 43*(12), 565–568.

Bernhard-Oettel, C., Isaksson, K., & Bellaagh, K. (2008). Patterns of contract motives and work involvement in temporary work: Relationships to work-related and general well-being. *Economic and Industrial Democracy, 29*(4), 565–591. https://doi.org/10.1177/0143831X08096231

Billings, D. (2004). Teaching learners from varied generations. *The Journal of Continuing Education in Nursing, 35*(3), 104–105.

Billings, D., & Kowalski, K. (2008). Developing your career as a nurse educator: The importance of having (or being) a mentor. *Journal of Continuing Education in Nursing, 39*(11), 490–491.

Bond, M. (2009) Exposing shame and its effect on clinical nursing education. *Journal of Nursing Education, 48*(3), 132–140.

Boud, D. (Ed.). (1988). *Developing student autonomy in learning.* Kogan Page.

Brown, T., Williams, B., McKenna, L., Palermo, C., McCall, L., Roller, L., Hewitt, L., Molloy, L., Baird, M., & Aldabah, L. (2011). Practice education learning environments: The mismatch between perceived and preferred expectations of undergraduate health science students. *Nurse Education Today, 31*, e22–e28. https://doi.org/10.1016/j.nedt.2010.11.013

Buccieri, K., Pivko, S., & Olzenak, D. (2013). Development of an expert clinical instructor: A theoretical model for clinical teaching in physical therapy. *Journal of Physical Therapy Education, 27*(1), 48–57.

Buruss, N., & Popkess, A. (2012). The diverse learning needs of students. In D. M. Billings & J. A. Halstead (Eds.), *Teaching in nursing: A guide for faculty* (4th ed., pp. 15–33). Elsevier Saunders.

Cederbaum, J., & Klusaritz, H. (2009). Clinical instruction: Using the strengths-based approach with nursing students. *Journal of Nursing Education, 48*(8), 422–428.

Center for Research on Teaching and Learning. (2014). *Guidelines for evaluating teaching.* University of Michigan. http://www.crlt.umich.edu/tstrategies/guidelines

Chally, p. (1992). Empowerment through teaching. *Journal of Nursing Education, 31*(3), 117–120.

Chan, D. (2001). Combining qualitative and quantitative methods in assessing hospital learning environments. *International Journal of Nursing Studies, 38*(4), 447–459.

Chan, D. (2002). Development of the clinical learning environment inventory: Using the theoretical framework of learning environment studies to assess nursing students' perceptions of the hospital as a learning environment. *Journal of Nursing Education, 41*(2), 69–75.

Chan, D. (2003). Validation of the clinical learning environment inventory. *Western Journal of Nursing Research, 25*(5), 519–532.

Chan, D. S. (2004). Nursing students' perception of hospital learning environments—An Australian perspective. *International Journal of Nursing Education Scholarship, 1*(1), 1–13.

Charfauros, K. H., & Tierney, W. G. (1999). Part-time faculty in colleges and universities: Trends and challenges in a turbulent environment. *Journal of Personnel Evaluation in Education, 13*(2), 141–151.

Child, J., & Langford, E. (2011). Exploring the learning experiences of nursing students with dyslexia. *Nursing Standard, 25*(40), 39–46.

Chitsabesan, P., Corbett, S., Walker, L., Spencer, J., & Barton, J. (2006). Describing clinical teachers' characteristics and behaviours using critical incidents and repertory grids. *Medical Education, 40,* 645–653.

Cook, L. (2005). Inviting teaching behaviours of clinical faculty and nursing students' anxiety. *Journal of Nursing Education, 44*(4), 156–161.

Courtney-Pratt, H., FitzGerald, M., Ford, K., Marsden, K., & Marlow, A. (2011). Quality clinical placements for undergraduate nursing students: A cross-sectional survey of undergraduates and supervising nurses. *Journal of Advanced Nursing, 68*(6), 1380–1390. https://doi.org/10.1111/j.1365-2648.2011.05851.x

Cross, T., Bazron, B., Dennis, K., & Isaacs, M. (1989). *Towards a culturally competent . system of care: A monograph on effective services for minority children who are severely emotionally disturbed.* Georgetown University Child Development Center, CASSP Technical Assistance Center.

Crouch, T. A. (2019). Perceptions of the possible impact of dyslexia on nursing and midwifery students and of the coping strategies they develop and/or use to help them cope in clinical practice. *Nurse Education in Practice, 35,* 90–97. https://doi.org/10.1016/j.nepr.2018.12.008

Curtis, J., Bowen, I., & Reid, A. (2007). You have no credibility: Nursing students' experiences of horizontal violence. *Nurse Education in Practice, 7*(3), 156–163.

Curtis, E., Jones, R., Tipene-Leach, D., Walker, C., Loring, B., Paine, S., & Reid, p. (2019). Why cultural safety rather than cultural competency is required to achieve health equity: A literature review and recommended definition. *International Journal for Equity in Health, 18*, Art. 174. https://doi.org/10.1186/s12939-019-1082-3

Davies, E. (1993). Clinical role modelling: Uncovering hidden knowledge. *Journal of Advanced Nursing, 18*, 627–636.

Dempsey, L. M. (2007). The experiences of Irish nurse lecturers' role transition from clinician to educator. *International Journal of Nursing Education Scholarship, 4*(1), 1–12.

Diekelmann, N. (2003). *Teaching the practitioners of care: New pedagogies for the health professions.* University of Wisconsin Press.

Dietitians of Canada. (n.d.). *Internships and practicum programs* [Fact sheet]. http://www.dietitians.ca/Career/Internships-Practicum-Programs/Overview.aspx

Duffy, A. (2009). Guiding students through reflective practice—The preceptors' experiences: A qualitative descriptive study. *Nurse Education in Practice, 9*(3), 166–175.

Dunn, S. V., & Burnett, p. (1995). The development of a clinical learning environment scale. *Journal of Advanced Nursing, 22*, 1166–1173.

Earle, V., & Myrick, F. (2009). Nursing pedagogy and the intergenerational discourse. *Journal of Nursing Education, 48*(11), 624–630. https://doi.org/10.3928/01484834-20090716-08

Fong, C., & McCauley, G. (1993). Measuring the nursing, teaching and interpersonal effectiveness of clinical instructors. *Journal of Nursing Education, 37*(7), 325–328.

Forneris, S. G., & Peden-McAlpine, C. (2009). Creating context for critical thinking in practice: The role of the preceptor. *Journal of Advanced Nursing, 65*(8), 1715–1724.

Franklin, N. (2010). Clinical supervision in undergraduate nursing students: A review of the literature. *E-Journal of Business Education & Scholarship of Teaching, 4*(1), 34–42.

Fry, B. (2011). *A nurse's guide to intergenerational diversity.* The Canadian Federation of Nurses Unions.

Gaberson, K., & Oermann, M. (2010). *Clinical teaching strategies in nursing* (3rd ed.). New York, NY: Springer.

Gappa, J. M. (2008). Today's majority: Faculty outside the tenure system. *Change: The Magazine of Higher Learning, 40*(4), 50–54. https://doi.org/10.3200/CHNG.40.4.50-54

Garneau, A. B., & Pepin, J. (2015). Cultural competence: A constructivist definition. *Journal of Transcultural Nursing, 26*(1), 9–15. https://doi.org/10.1177/1043659614541294

Gibson, S. (2009). Enhancing intergenerational communication in the classroom: Recommendations for successful teacher-student relationships. *Nursing Education Perspectives, 30*(1), 37–39.

Goethe, J. (1853/2013). *Goethe's opinions on the world, mankind, literature, science, and art*. Norderstedt, Germany: Books on Demand.

Griscti, O., Jacono, B., & Jacono, J. (2005). The nurse educator's clinical role. *Journal of Advanced Nursing, 50*(1), 84–92.

Guerra, O., & Kurtz, D. (2016). Building collaboration: A scoping review of cultural competency and safety education and training for healthcare students and professionals in Canada. *Teaching and Learning in Medicine, 29*(2), 129–142. https://doi.org/10.1080/10401334.2016.1234960

Guest, D. (2004). Flexible employment contracts, the psychological contract and employee outcomes: An analysis and review of the evidence. *International Journal of Management Review, 5–6*(1), 1–19.

Hampton, D., Welsh, D., & Wiggins, A. (2020). Learning preferences and engagement level of Generation Z nursing students. *Nurse Educator, 45*(3), 160–164. https://doi.org/10.1097/NNE.0000000000000710

Hand, H. (2006). Promoting effective teaching and learning in the clinical setting. *Nursing Standard, 20*(39), 55–63.

Hartigan-Rogers, J., Cobbett, S., Amirault, M., & Muise-Davis, M. (2007). Nursing graduates' perceptions of their undergraduate clinical placement. *International Journal of Nursing Education Scholarship, 4*, 1–12.

Hayajneh, F. (2011). Role model clinical instructor as perceived by Jordanian nursing students. *Journal of Research in Nursing, 16*(1), 23–32. https://doi.org/10.1177/1744987110364326

Heathcote, V. & Green, J. (2021). Transitioning from registered nurse to clinical nurse educator in the year of the nurse and midwife. *Journal of Nursing Education and Practice, 11*(4), 52–61. https://doi.org/10.5430/jnep.v11n4p52

Henderson, A., Cooke, M., Creedy, D., & Walker, R. (2012). Nursing students' perceptions of learning in practice environments: A review. *Nurse Education Today, 32*, 299–302. https://doi.org/10.1016/j.nedt.2011.03.010

Hickey, M. (2010). Baccalaureate nursing graduates' perceptions of their clinical instructional experiences and preparation for practice. *Journal of Professional Nursing, 26*(1), 35–41. https://doi.org/10.1016/j.profnurs.2009.03.001

Hill, K. S. (2004). Defy the decades with multigenerational teams. *Nursing Management, 35*(1), 32–35.

Holec, H. (1981). *Autonomy in foreign language learning*. Pergamon.

Howlin, F., Halligan, P., & O'Toole, S. (2014). Evaluation of a clinical needs assessment and exploration of the associated supports for students with a disability in clinical practice: Part 2. *Nurse Education in Practice, 14*(5), 565–572. https://doi.org/10.1016/j.nepr.2014.06.009

Jackson, D., Peters, K., Andrew, S., Salamonson, Y., & Halcomb, E. J. (2011). "If you haven't got a PhD, you're not going to get a job": The PhD as a hurdle to continuing academic employment in nursing. *Nurse Education Today, 31*, 340–344. https://doi.org/10.1016/j.nedt.2010.07.002

Jahangiri, L., McAndrew, M., Muzaffar, A., & Mucciolo, T. W. (2013). Characteristics of effective clinical teachers identified by dental students: A qualitative study. *European Journal of Dental Education, 17,* 10–18. https://doi.org/10.1111/eje.12012

Janssen, A. L., Macleod, R. D., & Walker, S. T. (2008). Recognition, reflection, and role models: Critical elements in education about care in medicine. *Palliative and Supportive Care, 6,* 389–395. https://doi.org/10.1017/S1478951508000618

Jetha, F., Boschma, G., & Clauson, M. (2016). Professional development needs of novice nursing instructors: A rapid evidence assessment. *International Journal of Nursing Education Scholarship, 13*(1), 1–10.

Johnson, S., & Romanello, M. (2005). Generational diversity: Teaching and learning approaches. *Nurse Educator, 30*(5), 212–216.

Jongen, C., McCalman, J., & Bainbridge, R. (2018). Health workforce cultural competency interventions: A systemic scoping review. *BMC Health Services Research, 18,* Art. 232. https://doi.org/10.1186/s12913-018-3001-5

Kelly, C. (2007). Students' perceptions of effective clinical teaching revisited. *Nurse Education Today, 27*(8), 885–892.

Kerka, S. (2000). Incidental learning (*Trends and Issues Alert, 18*). ERIC. http://www.calpro-online.org/eric/docs/tia00086.pdf

Kingston, A. (2014). Get ready for Generation Z. *Maclean's, 127*(28), 42–45.

Knowles, M. S. (1975). *Self-directed learning: A guide for learners and teachers.* Association Press.

Koontz, A., Mallory, J., Burns, J., & Chapman, S. (2010). Staff nurses and students: The good, the bad, and the ugly. *MEDSURG Nursing, 19*(4), 240–246.

Krueger, J. (2013). Pharmacy students' application of knowledge from the classroom to introductory pharmacy practice experiences. *American Journal of Pharmaceutical Education, 77*(2), Art. 31. https://doi.org/10.5688/ajpe77231

Kruse, S., Rakha, S., & Calderone, S. (2018). Developing cultural competency in higher education: An agenda for practice. *Teaching in Higher Education, 23*(6), 733–750. https://doi.org/10.1080/13562517.2017.1414790

Leaver, D. (2012). Clinical teaching skills for radiation therapy. *Radiation Therapist, 21*(2), 157–181.

L'Ecuyer, K. (2019a). Clinical education of nursing students with learning difficulties: An integrative review (part 1). *Nurse Education in Practice, 34,* 173–184.

L'Ecuyer, K. (2019b). Perceptions of nurse preceptors of students and new graduates with learning difficulties and their willingness to precept them in clinical practice (part 2). *Nurse Education in Practice, 34,* 210–217.

Levett-Jones, T., Higgins, I., & McMillan, M. (2009). Staff–student relationships and their impact on nursing students' belongingness and learning. *Journal of Advanced Nursing, 65*(2), 316–324.

Levett-Jones, T., Lathlean, J., Higgins, I., & McMillan M. (2008). The duration of clinical placements: A key influence on nursing students' experience of belongingness. *Australian Journal of Advanced Nursing, 26*(2), 8–16.

Little, D. (1991). *Learner autonomy I: Definitions, issues and problems.* Authentik.

Little, M., & Milliken, P. J. (2007). Practicing what we preach: Balancing teaching and clinical practice competencies. *International Journal of Nursing Education Scholarship, 4*(1), 1–14.

Marsick, V., & Watkins, K. (1990). *Informal and incidental learning in the workplace.* Routledge.

Marsick, V., & Watkins, K. (2001). Informal and incidental learning. *New Directions for Adult and Continuing Education, 89,* 25–34.

Masunaga, H., & Hitchcock, M. (2011). Aligning teaching practices with an understanding of quality teaching: A faculty development agenda. *Medical Teacher, 33,* 124–130.

McCall, L., Wray, N., & Lord, B. (2009). Factors affecting the education of pre-employment paramedic students during the clinical practicum. *Journal of Emergency Primary Health Care, 7*(4), Art. 990334. https://doi.org/10.33151/ajp.7.4.189

McCallum, C., Mosher, P., Jacobson, P., Gallivan, S., & Giuffre, S. (2013). Quality in physical therapist clinical education: A systematic review. *Physical Therapy, 93*(10), 1298–1311.

McCrindle, M., & Wolfinger, E. (2014). *The ABC of XYZ: Understanding the global generations.* McCrindle Research.

McCurry, M., & Martins, D. (2010). Teaching undergraduate nursing research: A comparison of traditional and innovative approaches for success with millennial learners. *Journal of Nursing Education, 49*(5), 276–279. https://doi.org/10.3928/01484834-20091217-02

McDermid, F., Peters, K., Daly, J., & Jackson, D. (2013). "I thought I was just going to teach": Stories of new nurse academics on transitioning from sessional teaching to continuing academic positions. *Contemporary Nurse, 45*(1), 46–55.

McPheat, C. (2014). Experience of nursing students with dyslexia on clinical placement. *Nursing Standard, 28*(41), 44–49.

Megivern, D., Pellerito, C., & Mowbray, C. (2003). Barriers to higher education for individuals with psychiatric disabilities. *Psychiatric Rehabilitation Journal, 26*(3), 217–232.

Meixner, C., Kruck, S. E., & Madden, L. T. (2010). Inclusion of part-time faculty for the benefit of faculty and students. *College Teaching, 58,* 141–147. https://doi.org/10.1080/87567555.2010.484032

Meloy, F., & Gambescia, S. F. (2014). Guidelines for response to student requests for academic considerations: Support versus enabling. *Nurse Educator, 39*(3), 138–142. https://doi.org/10.1097/NNE.0000000000000037

Melrose, S. (2004). What works? A personal account of clinical teaching strategies in nursing. *Education for Health, 17*(2), 236–239.

Melrose, S., Park, C., & Perry, B. (2020). *Centring human connections in the education of health professionals.* Athabasca University Press.

Melrose, S., & Shapiro, B. (1999). Students' perceptions of their psychiatric mental health clinical nursing experience: A personal construct theory exploration. *Journal of Advanced Nursing, 30*(6), 1451–1458.

Melrose, S., & Wishart, p. (2013). Resisting, reaching out and re-imagining to independence: LPNs' transitioning towards BNs and beyond. *International Journal of Nursing Education Scholarship, 10*(1), 1–7.

Mohammadi, E., Shahsavari, H., Mirzazadeh, A., Sohrabpour, A. A., & Mortaz Hejri, S. (2020). Improving role modeling in clinical teachers: A narrative literature review. *Journal of Advances in Medical Education & Professionalism, 8*(1), 1–9. https://doi.org/10.30476/jamp.2019.74929

Mohide, E., & Matthew-Maich, N. (2007). Implementation forum: Engaging nursing preceptor-student dyads in an evidence-based approach to professional practice. *Evidence-Based Nursing, 10*(2), 36–40.

Monroe, T., & Kenaga, H. (2010). Don't ask don't tell: Substance abuse and addiction among nurses. *Journal of Clinical Nursing, 20*, 504–509. https://doi.org/10.1111/j.1365-2702.2010.03518.x

Morris, D., & Turnbull, p. (2006). Clinical experiences of students with dyslexia. *Journal of Advanced Nursing, 54*(2), 238–247.

Mosca, C. (2019). The relationship between emotional intelligence and clinical teaching effectiveness. *Teaching and Learning in Nursing, 14*(2), 97–102. https://doi.org/10.1016/j.teln.2018.12.009

Murphy-Parker, D. (2013). Implementing policy for substance-related disorders in schools of nursing: The right thing to do. *Dean's Notes, 3*(4), 1–5.

Newton, M., Jolly, B., Ockerby, C., & Cross, W. (2010). Clinical Learning Environment Inventory: Factor analysis. *Journal of Advanced Nursing, 66*(6), 1371–1381. https://doi.org/10.1111/j.1365-2648.2010.05303.x

Notarianni, M., Curry-Lourenco, K., Barham, P., & Palmer, K. (2009). Engaging learners across generations: The progressive professional development model. *The Journal of Continuing Education in Nursing, 40*(6), 261–266. https://doi.org/10.9999/00220124-20090522

O'Connor, A. (2006). *Clinical instruction and evaluation: A teaching resource.* Jones & Bartlett.

Okoronkwo, I., Onyia-Pat, J., Agbo, M., Okpala, P., & Ndu, A. (2013). Students' perception of effective clinical teaching and teacher behaviour. *Open Journal of Nursing, 3*, 63–70. https://doi.org/10.4236/ojn.2013.31008

Parsh, B. (2010). Characteristics of effective simulated clinical experience instructors: Interviews with undergraduate nursing students. *Journal of Nursing Education, 49*(10), 569–572.

Paulis, M. (2011). Comparison of dental hygiene clinical instructor and student opinions of professional preparation for clinical instruction. *Journal of Dental Hygiene, 85*(4), 297–305.

Penn, B., Wilson, L., & Rosseter, R. (2008). Transitioning from nursing practice to a teaching role. *The Online Journal of Issues in Nursing, 13*(3), Ms. 3. https://doi.org/10.3912/OJIN.Vol13No03Man03

Perry, B. (2009). Role modeling excellence in clinical nursing practice. *Nurse Education in Practice, 9*, 36–44. https://doi.org/10.1016/j.nepr.2008.05.001

Puplampu, K. p. (2004). The restructuring of higher education and part-time instructors: A theoretical and political analysis of undergraduate teaching in Canada. *Teaching in Higher Education, 9*(2), 171–182. https://doi.org/10.1080/13562510420001953761

Rajagopal, I. (2004). Tenuous ties: The limited-term full-time faculty in Canadian universities. *Review of Higher Education, 28*(1), 49–75.

Ridley, C. (2011). The experiences of nursing students with dyslexia. *Nursing Standard, 25*, 24, 35–42.

Robinson, A. L., Andrews-Hall, S., & Fassett, M. (2007). Living on the edge: Issues that undermine the capacity of residential aged care providers to support student nurses on clinical placement. *Australian Health Review, 31*(3), 368–378.

Robinson, C. (2009). Teaching and clinical educator competency: Bringing two worlds together. *International Journal of Nursing Education Scholarship, 6*(1), Art. 20. https://doi.org/10.2202/1548-923X.1793

Rodger, K. (2019). Learning to think like a clinical teacher. *Teaching and Learning, 4*(1), 1–6. https://doi.org/10.1016/j.teln.2018.08.001

Rodger, S., Fitzgerald, C., Davila, W., Millar, F., & Allison, H. (2011). What makes a quality occupational therapy practice placement? Students' and practice educators' perspectives. *Australian Occupational Health Journal, 58*, 195–202.

Roger, S., Webb, G., Devitt, L., Gilbert, J., & Wrightson, p. (2008). Clinical education and practice placements in the allied health professions: An international perspective. *Journal of Allied Health, 37*(1), 53–62.

Ruesseler, M., & Obertacke, U. (2011). Teaching in daily clinical practice: How to teach in a clinical setting. *European Journal of Trauma Surgery, 37*, 313–316.

Sabog, R., Caranto, L., & David, J. (2015). Effective characteristics of a clinical instructor as perceived by BSU student nurses. *International Journal of Nursing Science, 5*(1), 5–19. http://article.sapub.org/10.5923.j.nursing.20150501.02.html

Salamonson, Y., Bourgeois, S., Everett, B., Weaver, R., Peters, K., & Jackson, D. (2011). Psychometric testing of the abbreviated Clinical Learning Environment Inventory (CLEI-19). *Journal of Advanced Nursing, 67*(12), 2668–2676. https://doi.org/10.1111/j.1365-2648.2011.05704.x

Sanderson-Mann, J., Wharrad, H., & McCandless, F. (2012). An empirical exploration of the impact of dyslexia on placement-based learning, and a comparison with non-dyslexic students. *Diversity and Equality in Health and Care, 9*, 89–99.

Schmutz, A., Gardner-Lubbe, S., & Archer, E. (2013). Clinical educators' self-reported personal and professional development after completing a short course in undergraduate clinical supervision at Stellenbosch University. *African Journal of Health Professions Education, 5*(1), 8–13. https://doi.org/10.7196/AJHPE.194

Sherman, R. (2009). Teaching the net set. *Journal of Nursing Education, 48*(7), 359–360. https://doi.org/10.3928/01484834-20090615

Sieh, S., & Bell, S. (1994). Perceptions of effective clinical teachers in associate degree programs. *Journal of Nursing Education, 33*(9), 389–394.

Smedley, B., Stith, A., & Nelson, A. (2003). *Unequal treatment: Confronting racial and ethnic disparities in health care*. National Academies Press.

Smith, C., Swain, A., & Penprase, B. (2011). Congruence of perceived effective clinical teaching characteristics between students and preceptors of nurse anesthesia programs. *Journal of the American Association of Nurse Anesthetists, 79*(4), 62–68.

Smith, L. (2018). A nurse educator's guide to cultural competence. *Nursing Made Incredibly Easy, 16*(2), 19–23. https://doi.org/10.1097/01.NME.0000529955.66161.1e

Sonn, I., & Vermeulen, N. (2018). Occupational therapy students' experiences and perceptions of culture during fieldwork. *South African Journal of Occupational Therapy, 48*(1), 34–39. https://doi.org/10.17159/2310-3833/2017/vol48n1a7

Sparks & Honey. (n.d.). *Meet Generation Z: Forget everything you learned about millennials* [Power Point]. http://www.slideshare.net/sparksandhoney/generation-z-final-june-17

Stewart, A., & Torges, C. (2006). Social, historical and developmental influences on the psychology of the Baby Boom at midlife. In S. Whitbourne & S. L. Willis (Eds.), *The Baby Boomers grow up: Contemporary perspectives on midlife* (pp. 23–43). Lawrence Erlbaum Associates.

Storrie, K., Ahern, K., & Tuckett, A. (2012). Crying in the halls: Supervising students with symptoms of emotional problems in the clinical practicum. *Teaching in Higher Education, 17*(1), 89–103.

Tanner, C. (2006). The next transformation: Clinical education. *Journal of Nursing Education, 45*, 99–100.

Tilka Miller, E. (2007). Bridging the generation gap. *Rehabilitation Nursing, 32*(1), 2–3, 43.

Walker, J. T., Martin, T., White, J., & Elliot, R. (2006). Generational (age) differences in nursing students' preferences for teaching methods. *Journal of Nursing Education, 45*(9), 371–376.

Weston, M. (2006). Integrating generational perspectives in nursing. *Online Journal of Issues in Nursing, 11*(2), 2.

Williams, C. (2019). Nurse educators meet your new students: Generation Z. *Nurse Educator, 44*(2), 59–60. https://doi.org/10.1097/NNE.0000000000000637

Wortsman, A., & Crupi, A. (2009). *Addressing issues of intergenerational diversity in the nursing workplace*. Canadian Federation of Nurses Unions.

Wray, J., Aspland, J., Taghzouit, J., & Pace, K. (2013). Making the nursing curriculum more inclusive for students with specific learning difficulties (SpLD): Embedding specialist study skills into a core module. *Nurse Education Today, 33*, 602–607.

4

Maintaining Resilience through Positive Collaborations

I am a teacher at heart, and there are moments when I can hardly hold the joy. When my students and I discover uncharted territory to explore, when the pathway out of a thicket opens up before us, when our experience is illumined by the lightening-life of the mind— then teaching is the finest work I know.

PARKER PALMER (2007, P. 1)

As Parker Palmer so eloquently wrote, teaching can be joyful, illuminating, and fine work that involves exploring the world through the eyes of our learners. Yet, for educators in clinical settings, negative influences on learning can sometimes seem to be beyond their control. Such influences can hamper the joyful potential of the educational experience for both educators and learners. As we have emphasized throughout this book, learning in unpredictable clinical environments presents distractions and challenges that are different from those that students face in traditional classrooms. Collaborating with learners to support their success in clinical placement experiences poses unique challenges for educators. Still, the intense satisfaction that educators and learners alike feel when new skills are mastered, new knowledge is assimilated, and new attitudes emerge is universal. Achieving these accomplishments (and the sense of joy that Parker describes) requires multiple approaches among educators, including skills founded on effective learner-teacher collaboration.

The challenges that learners face in clinical environments are those that they will face in practice after graduation. When clinical teachers guide learners toward developing positive and collaborative ways of managing these challenges, they provide them with vital skills on which they can continue to build throughout their careers. These skills are essential for health-care providers if they are to remain resilient and continue to do their work successfully. Consistently providing compassionate care to patients or clients and their families over extended periods of time and under difficult circumstances can take a toll on health-care professionals. The work can be emotionally demanding and mentally exhausting and leave health-care providers feeling isolated and exhausted.

Typically, teaching approaches in clinical settings focus on helping learners to acquire the physical skills that they need to provide competent evidence-informed care. Yet neglecting to acknowledge that emotional demands exist in the practice setting, and that strategies are available to ameliorate these demands, is shortsighted. Essentially, if clinical teachers hope to guide learners through the "uncharted territory" to which Palmer refers, then they must help learners to develop and sustain feelings of joy and passion for their chosen profession. In our view, actions that support learners in developing this capacity are grounded in a positive frame of reference that recognizes the cost of caring and embraces a commitment to enhancing emotional resilience. Clinical teachers must also invite learners to consider the impacts that meaningful collaborations with others can have on promoting and strengthening their own emotional health and well-being. In this chapter, we invite clinical teachers to consider how positive collaborations and relationships can foster their success as educators while keeping them healthy and able to continue the important work of teaching health-care providers.

RECOGNIZING THE COST OF CARING

Providing compassionate care to patients/clients when they are at their most vulnerable can be physically and emotionally demanding for health-care professionals. Helping and caring for others involve a high degree of altruism. Although work in the helping professions provides limitless opportunities for satisfaction and personal growth, it can come at a personal cost. The extent to which skilful "self-giving" is required can cause suffering for caregivers (McAllister & McKinnon, 2009). When health-care professionals engage in self-giving, they might attend to the needs of others at the expense of taking care of their own physical and emotional needs. Carers might neglect their own health and view self-care as a low priority (Foureur et al., 2013).

Experiences of feeling burned out are common. The word *burnout* was initially defined as "a syndrome of emotional exhaustion, depersonalisation, and reduced personal accomplishment that can occur among individuals who work with people in some capacity" (Maslach et al., 1996, p. 4). In response to feeling burned out, people distance themselves emotionally as a form of self-protection (Maslach et al., 1996). The World Health Organization (2018) extended this seminal definition to emphasize that burnout also includes feelings of negativism or cynicism related to one's job. Learners in clinical environments can expect to encounter health-care professionals who are experiencing some, if not all, of the negative emotions associated with burnout. For example, in a cross-sectional survey of nurses from 12 countries in Europe and the United States, 42% of the nurses described themselves as "burned out" (Aiken et al., 2012).

According to Grant and Kinman (2014), the emotionally demanding nature of work in health-care fields can also lead to secondary trauma (emotional distress associated with hearing about the first-hand trauma experienced by another), vicarious trauma (a damaging shift in beliefs about the world in response to being repeatedly exposed to traumatic material), and compassion fatigue (physical, mental, and emotional withdrawal associated with caring for sick or traumatized people especially if you are not able to relieve their suffering). Health-care professionals frequently experience psychological distress in relation to their role, the wider organizational context, a perceived lack of control, and interactions with patients/clients that evoke strong emotional reactions (Grant & Kinman, 2014).

Although compassion fatigue is a syndrome usually associated with the negative effects of providing care to the ill, there is emerging evidence that educators can experience a similar syndrome as they care about the success of students and come to know of stress and suffering among students that they are unable to relieve. Educators can be vulnerable to compassion fatigue since the teaching profession attracts individuals who gain satisfaction in caring for people (Krop, 2013; Showalter, 2010). Many who enter teaching as a profession are empathetic and nurturing individuals "whose personal identity is closely associated with their professional role" (Boyle, 2011, p. 1; Fowler, 2015; Hunsaker et al., 2015; Krop, 2013). Caring is often viewed as a fundamental value of the teaching profession. Educators might see their students' success as their own in some ways (Isenbarger & Zembylas, 2006) and often come to care about the success and well-being of learners. Teachers can experience emotional labour as they teach, nurture, and guide individuals along their life paths for sustained periods of time, often years (Isenbarger & Zembylas, 2006). These factors make educators—especially those who genuinely care about their learners and aim to get to know them well—at risk of compassion fatigue.

The cost of caring is not limited to practising health-care professionals and educators. Learners can experience similar negative emotions. They can have strong emotional reactions to clinical placements, they can feel conflicted between their role as a learner and their role as an emerging professional, and they can perceive themselves as ineffective (Grant & Kinman, 2014). Many health-care learners experience feelings of depression (Rakesh et al., 2017). Learners are often reluctant to disclose that they are experiencing difficulties, exacerbating potentially damaging negative emotions (Grant & Kinman, 2014).

Like practitioners and learners, educators in health fields are also affected by the cost of caring. People who work in most areas of education are considered helping professionals, and they often give generously of themselves in their work with learners. Educators have frequently expressed that they feel extremely stressed (Thomas et al., 2019), overwhelmed by emotional demands, and as though they are merely surviving rather than thriving (Aguilar, 2018).

Given that clinical teachers straddle the fields of both health and education, they can expect to face ongoing personal challenges related to their own emotional health throughout their careers. At times, emotional depletion and negativity can distract from a view of teaching as fulfilling, enjoyable, and satisfying work. When educators in health fields do view their teaching as satisfying, they are more likely to do their work in an exemplary way (Melrose et al., 2020). An important first step that clinical teachers can take toward feeling less depleted and more fulfilled is intentionally to articulate the positive aspects of clinical teaching that are especially meaningful to them.

A Strategy to Try ▶ *What I Love Most about Clinical Teaching Is. . . .*
When you are feeling relaxed and in a comfortable setting, take a few moments to reflect deeply on what you love most about clinical teaching. Think about the times when you have genuinely experienced joy and fulfillment from your teaching. Record your response(s) on a sticky note and post it somewhere visible.

If you find this strategy meaningful, you might wish to implement it with your learners. Simply change the question to "What I love most about [my profession] is. . . ."

EMOTIONAL LABOUR

The cost of caring is further illustrated with an explanation of the term "emotional labour." It refers to the process by which workers are expected to manage their feelings in accordance with organizationally defined rules and guidelines (Hochschild, 1983/2003). Emotional labour affects people who work in areas where there is intensive contact with the public and where people are expected to regulate their emotions during interactions with others (Hochschild, 1983/2003). Some workplace roles (including those in health and education fields) stipulate either formally or informally that certain emotions can be displayed publicly, whereas others are expected to be kept private. For example, expressing patience and empathy is considered appropriate, whereas showing frustration and disgust is not (Kinman & Leggetter, 2016).

Daily, health-care practitioners, learners, and clinical teachers all engage in emotionally charged contacts with patients/clients. In addition to those intense contacts, learners engage in equally intense interactions with practitioners and their clinical teachers, especially during evaluation activities. Certainly, appropriate responses are expected in public. Yet powerful emotions that are not considered appropriate to display are also present. The emotional labour expected of professionals requires that these emotions remain private. It is important to note that the notion of "private" does not mean that these emotions are to remain unacknowledged. Rather, it emphasizes the importance of finding suitable outlets for expressing certain emotions.

When people continue to work and learn in situations in which their need for emotional expression does not conform to workplace expectations of emotional labour (whether real or perceived), they can experience profound emotional strain and dissonance (Kinman & Leggetter, 2016). The effort required to keep emotions hidden below the surface and act well emotionally drains people of their emotional resources and leaves them feeling stressed, conflicted, depleted, mentally exhausted, and burned out (Delgado et al., 2017; Kinman & Leggetter, 2016). It adversely affects workplace interactions, workplace relationships, and ultimately workplace performance (Delgado et al., 2020). For those with limited experience in a caring role, navigating the demands of emotional labour inherent in the role of health-care professional can be particularly problematic (Kinman & Leggetter, 2016).

Believing that emotional regulation requires people to suppress their emotions is not healthy. Although health-care professionals would encourage their patients/clients to find respectful and appropriate ways to express their emotions (even those construed as negative), opportunities to do so might not be immediately available to the professionals themselves. As educators, it is critical to assess expectations related to emotional labour in the clinical settings in which students are learning. The rules and guidelines might be more implicit than explicit. Expressions of emotions that are viewed as inappropriate in one setting might be quite different in another. Not all members of staff groups will model healthy regulation of their emotions.

Recognizing and acknowledging that emotional labour (the ability to regulate emotions) is expected in professional fields is an important foundational step in helping learners to prepare for the realities of practice. Aspects of the topic are often addressed under curriculum concepts related to "professionalism." To be fully informative, however, clinical teachers must instigate discussions of how to manage (and importantly to express) the negative feelings and responses that professionals inevitably experience in practice settings.

Health professionals are expected to regulate their emotions (known as emotional labour). Some positive emotions (e.g., compassion) may be displayed publicly, whereas others (e.g., revulsion) are considered negative and expected to be kept private. Regulating emotions does not mean suppressing or denying them. Educators can pay more attention to cultivating learners' capacities to express their positive emotions than to managing negative feelings.

Consider opportunities in which you could facilitate a discussion of negative emotions with learners. Begin by reflecting on your own experiences. Think about a time when you experienced an intense negative response in a patient care situation. You might have acted or wanted to act in ways that could be perceived as inappropriate. What might a healthy response look like? Which actions could you have taken, or did you take, that were appropriate and fitting for the situation?

With the goal of modelling healthy ways of expressing negative emotions, share your process of reflecting with learners.

ENHANCING EMOTIONAL RESILIENCE

As the preceding discussion emphasized, the caring and emotional labour required of health-care professionals, learners, and clinical teachers alike affect their emotional well-being. Consistently expressing positive rather than negative emotions, together with approaching stressful workplace challenges as opportunities rather than setbacks, require ongoing efforts. Positive emotions are more than just being happy; they reflect a deeper approach to how life is experienced (Pipe et al., 2012; Tugade et al., 2004). Emotions that express positivity are those rich in joy, gratitude, serenity, interest, hope, pride, amusement, inspiration, awe, and love (Fredrickson, 2009). People who can display these kinds of positive emotions, even under difficult circumstances, are viewed as emotionally resilient.

The word *resilience* is defined as "the process of adapting well in the face of adversity, trauma, tragedy, threats or even significant sources of stress" (American Psychological Association, 2014, para 4). Resilience is a multidimensional psychological construct that overlaps with other constructs, including organizational resilience and individual workplace resilience (Rees et al., 2015). Organizational resilience is an organization's or institution's ability and capacity to handle disruptive events (Ruiz-Martin et al., 2018). Individual resilience is an employee's ability to handle adversity successfully (Hartmann et al., 2020). Not unexpectedly, people who work in highly resilient organizations have more opportunities to learn about and develop their individual resilience. A strong, supportive, and team-oriented culture can help health-care professionals to manage the emotional demands of their roles (Cheng et al., 2013).

In health-care settings, clinical teachers might have limited control over the level of organizational resilience demonstrated in the clinical environments in which their students learn. A culture of coping dominated by negativity and emotional distancing might be present in these places. The role models that learners are exposed to might not handle the cost of caring well, and they might struggle with the demands of emotional labour that their roles require of them. However, clinical teachers do control the extent to which they demonstrate their own resilience and how they invite learners to do likewise. A dimension of resilience that is well suited to instruction in clinical areas is emotional resilience.

It refers to the element of affect that is inherent in resilience. Emotional resilience is the ability to "recover" from adversity, react appropriately, or "bounce back" when life gets tough (Grant & Kinman, 2014). When applied to health-care workplace settings, emotional resilience is further explained as the ability to maintain personal and professional well-being in the face of ongoing work stress and adversity (McCann et al., 2013). Health-care professionals who have enhanced emotional resilience express less negativity and feel less overwhelmed by job stresses (McCann et al., 2013; Stacey & Cook, 2019).

Emotional resilience, like all forms of resilience, is not an innate, fixed characteristic; rather, it is a skill that can be developed and enhanced (Grant & Kinman, 2014; Stephens, 2013). Research suggests that integrating educational content and instruction in resilience can help learners in the health-care professions to feel stronger, more focused, and better able to endure negative emotions (Grant & Kinman, 2014; McAllister & McKinnon, 2009; Stacey et al., 2017). For example, when resilience competencies were integrated into a nursing curriculum, students thought that the self-care interventions that they learned increased their ability to provide compassionate care to patients (Stacey et al., 2017). Similarly, when resilience-building activities were included in their curriculum, student physicians found that they were better able to empathize with patients, combat stress and burnout, and gain awareness of ways to promote a culture of mutual openness and understanding (Rakesh et al., 2017). Furthermore, introducing emotional resilience strategies to social work students helped them to deal with the emotional demands of their profession (Grant & Kinman, 2014).

A Strategy to Try ▶ *Inspiring Stories of People Who Are Emotionally Resilient* Some people have experienced devastating events in their lives, but they can "bounce back" with positivity and optimism. Emotionally resilient, they seem to be able to cope with and find pleasure in whatever comes their way. When you think of emotional resilience, does a specific person come to mind? Perhaps a family member or workplace mentor? A patient/ client who did not view her or his condition as a limitation? A historical figure or contemporary hero portrayed in the news? Jot down the story(ies) or find relevant video clips online and integrate them into information and educational content that you share with learners.

APPROACHES FOR ENHANCING EMOTIONAL RESILIENCE

In their research exploring emotional resilience in practising and student social workers, Grant and Kinman (2014) identified how people who were able to adapt positively to stressful working conditions (and manage their emotional demands) demonstrated four competencies that are helpful in training students to become resilient professionals: reflective ability, emotional intelligence, social confidence, and social support. None of these competencies can be achieved by learners on their own. Collaborations and connections with others are required. Next we explain how clinical teachers can create the kinds of collaborations that will help learners to enhance these competencies.

Reflective ability can be enhanced when learners are provided with opportunities to reflect on their practice, consider their personal motivations, and explore the nature and impact of their interactions with others. *Emotional intelligence* (with which people are able to persist in the face of frustration, control impulses, delay gratification, establish emotional boundaries, avoid overinvolvement with patients/clients, and "accurately" empathize with others) can be enhanced when learners are provided with safe spaces in which to discuss their emotional responses to distressing events. *Social confidence* (e.g., demonstrating assertiveness and conflict resolution skills) can be enhanced when learners are encouraged to challenge instances of poor clinical practice and share appropriately the negative emotions that these poor practices evoke. *Social support* can be enhanced when learners are consistently invited to connect in meaningful ways with their educators, preceptors/practitioners, and fellow students.

Grant and Kinman (2014) further posit that specific approaches to developing the competencies in emotional resilience mentioned above can be grouped into the categories of reflective practice, supervision, and peer coaching. Although these approaches can be included in health professions curricula in other topic areas, the specific links to enhancing emotional resilience might not be identified.

Reflective Practice

Reflective practice is familiar to most health-care professional practitioners and learners. Thinking about and reflecting on what went well, what could be improved, and how to incorporate needed changes are essential skills that should be implemented in everyday practice. When clinical teachers extend the reflective process to include an understanding of emotional resilience, they deepen learners' insights into regulating their own emotions. Inviting learners to reflect honestly and critically on their negative (as well as positive) feelings can create openings to explore appropriate ways of expressing rather than suppressing negative emotions.

A Strategy to Try ▶ *Write a Narrative from a Patient/Client's Perspective*
Grant and Kinman (2014) assert that writing a narrative from a patient/client's perspective can enhance emotional resilience in health-care profession learners. Have learners write a short narrative or account of an experience as though they were a patient/client. Alternatively, learners could express their narratives in the form of a poem.

Have learners share their narratives (or poems) with peers during small group discussions. Draw out reflections on emotional resilience. Invite discussion of examples in which negative emotions were displayed appropriately and inappropriately. Encourage participants to create links between the narratives and their own professional growth.

Supervision

Supervision, in the context of enhancing emotional resilience, refers to the interactions between educators and learners individually and in groups. The interactions might be when educators are observing learners performing skills, providing feedback on their performance, or drawing out their thinking during individual and group discussions. Because of the evaluative component clearly present in interactions in which educators are supervising learners, there is an imbalance of power.

This imbalance can create a barrier to the safe spaces needed for learners to disclose their negative emotions. Those emotions might not be fully recognized, they can be perceived as too shameful to express, or they might be directly related to the educator. However, positive role modelling can help to break down these barriers. In the many varied supervisory and interactive activities that educators engage in with learners, educators can demonstrate approaches that enhance emotional resilience, and they can comment intentionally on the strategies that have worked for them. They can also ensure that opportunities for connecting with like-minded others, such as fellow students, are also available to learners. The capacity to seek out (and engage in) supportive relationships is an essential component of resilience building, and it is an ability that learners will need throughout their practice (Grant & Kinman, 2014).

A Strategy to Try ▶ *One Strategy that I Use to Create a Safe Emotional Space Is....* When you supervise learners as they perform a skill, answer a question, or participate in a group discussion, identify one strategy that you use to create a feeling of emotional safety within the interaction. Given that educators evaluate learners, how do you intentionally invite learners to share their feelings (even the negative ones)? Are there opportunities to use this strategy more frequently? Might other strategies related to creating safe emotional spaces also be useful in your interactions with learners?

If you are part of a community of educators (e.g., part of a faculty at an educational institution), then consider including sharing teaching strategies (e.g., how to create safe emotional spaces for learners) during professional development sessions. In this way, the community can build a repertoire of successful approaches.

Peer Coaching/Mentoring

Peer coaching/mentoring can also help learners to enhance their emotional resilience and find ways to protect themselves against the negative effects of emotional labour (Grant & Kinman, 2014; Kinman and Leggetter, 2016). When the relationships are mutually supportive and reciprocal, learners can experience a sense of connection with others in similar circumstances. Peers can provide valuable emotional support to one another (Andersen & Watkins, 2018).

Typically, in most educational experiences, learners find peer relationships on their own. However, these relationships might not be focused directly on finding positive ways of coping with the emotional demands of practice. Institutions of higher learning can designate students to serve as peer coaches, mentors, tutors, or counsellors and give them basic training in order to provide emotional support; however, students, educators, and mentors all have different perspectives on a mentor's role and how it should be enacted (Colvin & Ashman, 2010). When students are in clinical settings and working alongside practitioners, they might not have access to these peers when they need the support. Often, moreover, the situations that they encounter involve patient/client or staff confidentiality and should not be discussed with people who are not directly involved in the situation, such as peer coaches.

Clinical teachers are uniquely positioned to design activities in which peers can focus on emotional resilience in their connections with one another. Having students work in pairs is an established educational strategy (e.g., a "study buddy" approach). Integrating a focus on enhancing resilience into this established strategy provides an opportunity for learners to acknowledge that negative emotions exist and to explore practical ways to express and cope with these emotions. This focus can also encourage learners to think about approaches that they can use to support their colleagues during emotionally stressful times, which are common in clinical practice.

Although the elements of mutual trust and genuine concern that are present in self-initiated peer relationships might never develop in assigned student partnership activities, the interactions can nonetheless open the door for discussion (and learning) that might not otherwise occur. Introducing role-playing activities to student pairs enables them to practise expressing and responding during emotionally charged interactions (Kinman and Leggetter, 2016).

A Strategy to Try ▶ *Role-Play an Emotionally Charged Professional Interaction (in Pairs)*

Assign a partner to each member of the learning group. Describe a situation that could arise in your clinical area in which a staff member might feel overwhelmed by a traumatic and distressing workplace incident. Instruct one student in each dyad to play the role of the staff member who feels overwhelmed and the other to play the role of an emotionally supportive colleague. After five minutes, have participants switch roles.

Follow the activity with a group discussion. Pose questions that invite reflection on the importance of expressing, rather than suppressing, negative emotions during collegial interactions. Encourage participants to share their perceptions of both appropriate and inappropriate displays of emotion.

CULTIVATING POSITIVE COLLABORATIONS

Beyond ensuring that supervisory activities with learners include safe spaces, and that peer coaching/mentoring opportunities are available to learners, clinical teachers can enhance emotional resilience by strategically finding ways to cultivate positive collaborations. The interpersonal connections so necessary for health-care professionals to develop and maintain a positive and resilient outlook on their practice might not just happen. In the following discussion, we comment on how promoting civility, harnessing anxiety, and resolving conflict in a positive way can support positive collaborations.

In all of their collaborations with patients/clients and members of health-care teams, health-care profession learners are expected to demonstrate and promote civil (polite, courteous, and respectful) behaviour. Everyone expects to be treated by those in clinical workplaces with civility. Unfortunately, reports from institutions across many sectors, including those that provide health-care services, indicate a rise in incivility (Craft et al., 2020; Pattani et al., 2018).

In workplace environments, incivility is defined as low-intensity behaviours in either words or gestures that can confer indirect harm on colleagues and cultivate a toxic work culture (Pattani et al., 2018). Examples of incivility include eye-rolling, bullying, verbal abuse or rudeness, excessive competitiveness, social exclusion, inaction (e.g., not responding to emails), and other forms of disrespect (Pattani et al., 2018). Some serious manifestations of incivility, such as physical abuse and sexual harassment, violate the law (Zhu et al., 2019). Despite indications that incivility has negatively affected organizational operating costs, employee turnover, employee performance, group cohesion, and organizational commitment in health care (as well as other industries), problems with incivility continue to emerge in many workplaces (Porath & Pearson, 2013).

In academic settings, the definition of incivility is extended to include the notion that behaviours that interfere with the learning process are also considered uncivil (Robertson, 2012). Incivility can be demonstrated by students toward faculty or other students and by faculty toward students, other faculty, or administration. Examples of student incivility in classrooms and labs include disrupting class, using cellphones or computers for activities not related to class, carrying on side conversations during class, making negative remarks, challenging instructors inappropriately, pressuring faculty to meet their demands (e.g., increasing a grade), and dominating discussions (i.e., preventing other students from joining in them). Outside the classroom, students who act with incivility can discredit faculty; complain about them; speak negatively about their program; gossip about other students; demand make-up assignments, extensions, or grade changes; and fail to follow the appropriate lines of communication (Clark & Carnosso, 2008; Clark & Springer, 2007; Penconek, 2014, 2020).

Examples of faculty incivility toward students include challenging students' knowledge in front of the class, belittling students in front of others, displaying favouritism, demonstrating inconsistency with evaluations, complaining about their profession, and not providing an open and secure forum for discussing concerns (Clark & Carnosso, 2008; Clark & Springer, 2007; Penconek, 2014). Faculty also demonstrate incivility when they arrive late for class, provide learners with unclear expectations, change or have a poorly constructed syllabus, or set a cold, unwelcoming, or disrespectful tone in the classroom or clinical setting (Robertson, 2012).

In clinical areas, examples of faculty and practitioner incivility include showing lack of professionalism in the workplace, being disrespectful and unfair toward students, and making students feel unwanted and ignored in the workplace (Zhu et al., 2019). When faculty behave in uncivil ways toward other faculty or administrators, they might refuse to answer questions, make condescending remarks or express "put-downs," indicate that they are unavailable, present a distant or cold demeanour, or exert rank or superiority (Clark & Carnosso, 2008).

When people in any setting experience incivility, they can leave the situation feeling highly distressed (Clark & Carnosso, 2008; Clark et al., 2009; Robertson, 2012). The negative feelings and emotional depletion can persist long after the incident has passed, making it difficult to remain emotionally resilient and find enjoyment in one's career. When health-care profession students experience incivility in their academic or clinical education, they can leave their programs or be acculturated to become uncivil professionals (Milesky et al., 2015). Educators who experience incivility suffer anxiety and poor performance, and they might leave academia altogether (Milesky et al., 2015).

When incivility is present in clinical environments, it can spread to academic environments and vice versa. Incivility leads to toxic work environments that adversely affect patients/clients (Layne et al., 2019; Milesky et al., 2015; Pattani et al., 2018; Pronovost & Vohr, 2010). Clearly, any effort that clinical teachers can make toward understanding possible triggers of incivility and finding ways to promote civility is time well spent. A significant relationship exists between unmanaged job stress/anxiety (including difficulty resolving conflicts) and incivility in the workplace (Oyeleye et al., 2013).

Definitions of civil behaviour, or behaviour that most people would consider polite, courteous, and respectful, can be articulated in different ways. It can seem to be easier to define incivility (behaviour that is not civil and includes words or gestures that can confer indirect harm on others). Think about what civility looks like in the clinical area in which you teach. How do the practitioners demonstrate (or do not demonstrate) their respect for one another, for students, and for you? How do you demonstrate respect to others in the workplace? Your observations will form a basis for your personal definition of civility.

Use your definition to set expectations of civil behaviour that you require of yourself and of your students. Once you have a clear view of civil behaviour, include a discussion of how learners perceive civil/uncivil behaviours. Have them draw up a "contract" and commit to enacting civility in their learning environments.

In the following discussion, we comment on how techniques geared to harnessing anxiety and resolving conflict can begin to help learners strengthen their emotional resilience and collaborate successfully with those whom they encounter in clinical settings.

HARNESSING ANXIETY

When practitioners, educators, and learners are burdened by heavy workloads, family responsibilities, and the emotional labour required of professionals, they can expect to feel anxiety at times. It can be displayed through inappropriate expressions of negative emotion and incivility. For learners, mild to moderate levels of anxiety can benefit learning, but high levels of anxiety result in decreased learning (Melincavage, 2011). High levels of anxiety in clinical environments can have profound impacts on learners' personal lives and on their clinical performance (Melo et al., 2010; Turner & McCarthy, 2016).

Just as teaching approaches that emphasize reflective practice, supervision that includes safe psychological spaces, and structured activities in which peer coaching/mentoring occur can enhance emotional resilience, so too these approaches can harness learner anxiety. Self-reflection techniques help learners to mediate stress, gain insight, and learn appropriate coping behaviours (Eng & Pai, 2015). Supervision by clinical teachers that invites learners to share their preferred learning styles and to articulate anxiety management strategies that have worked for them in the past will help to lower their levels of anxiety. Peer coaching/mentoring in clinical environments can decrease anxiety and confusion among students, increase their positive educational environments, improve their responsibility, promote their active learning, enhance their involvement, and help to develop their ability to mentor in the future (Sprengel & Job, 2004).

Additionally, as health professionals themselves, clinical teachers have a repertoire of anti-anxiety management techniques that are effective with patients/clients. Modelling these techniques during high-stress interactions with students can have a positive and far-reaching influence. One such technique, mindfulness, is gaining increasing recognition as a way of regulating negative emotions, including anxiety.

Mindfulness, in relation to health professionals' own emotional wellness, was initially conceptualized as a logical extension of the concept of reflective practice. Ronald Epstein (1999), a physician and leader in mindfulness techniques, defined mindfulness as a process of remaining present in everyday experiences and being open to all thoughts, actions, and sensations. This openness includes being cognizant of one's own mental processes, being aware of what is occurring around oneself, and responding with acts of compassion (Epstein, 1999). In short, mindfulness calls professionals to attend intentionally in an open and discerning way to whatever arises in the present moment (Shapiro, 2009).

A growing body of research links mindfulness techniques to enhanced emotional well-being, and calls for integrating mindfulness training as a self-care strategy into health professions education programs are increasing (Foureur et al., 2013; Irving et al., 2009; Reid, 2013). Learning institutions that offer programs for health-care professionals can integrate mindfulness techniques, resources, and practice sessions into the curriculum. In these instances, students bring this foundational knowledge from the classroom directly to their clinical practice. In other instances, learning institutions can offer workshops or individual training sessions on mindfulness through their student services or counselling centres. Additionally, health-care organizations and clinical agencies can provide mindfulness training through their human resources or employee assistance programs.

When clinical teachers are aware of resources related to mindfulness that are available to students, they can incorporate them into their clinical teaching and extend students' existing knowledge.

A Strategy to Try ▶ *Investigate Mindfulness Resources Available in Your Area*
Mindfulness, or remaining aware, open, and discerning regarding what is going on in the present moment, can strengthen people's feelings of positivity and lower their stress levels. Investigate whether any mindfulness training is available to your students through their curriculum, program, or clinical agency. Invite students to share what they know about mindfulness and encourage those who feel comfortable doing so to lead the group in a mindfulness exercise. Demonstrate any mindfulness techniques that have worked for you. Whenever possible, integrate the mindfulness training that students have been offered through their program.

From the Field ▶ *Centring to Become Fully Present*

Upon arrival in the clinical area, gather the group together in a quiet place (even the clean utility room). With gentle intonation, read or adapt the following script:

> Close your eyes or soften your gaze and breathe in and out. With each breath in, breathe in strength, hope, and possibility. With each breath out, let go of fears, preoccupations, and burdens in your life. As you breathe more deeply, notice the breath soften the belly, opening the heart, making way for your gifts to come to the surface. Notice your feet on the floor, rooted—you are supported. At any point today, you can return to the breath softening the belly, opening the heart.

MARY ANN MORRIS, RN, MSN, SELKIRK COLLEGE

RESOLVING CONFLICT

Conflict is inevitable in situations in which people must interact with one another in order to learn and work. Although professionals in the business fields have come to recognize conflict as a potential source of learning and innovation, professionals in the health fields still tend to view conflict through a negative lens, often considering it to be disruptive, inefficient, and unprofessional (Eichbaum, 2018). Consequently, many health professions practitioners and learners tend to avoid conflict or try to resolve it quickly.

When people disagree and argue, they are in conflict; however, when they reach an agreement, they are said to have resolved that conflict. Certainly, health-care professionals are not expected to resolve all disagreements. However, they are expected to engage in civil interactions that do not leave anyone involved feeling distressed and emotionally depleted. They can respectfully "agree to disagree."

There is a plethora of conflict resolution theories and models, and health professions programs can adapt a specific model that learners are expected to use when conflicts arise in their academic or clinical environments. The model can be framed more from a problem-solving orientation than from a focus on conflict resolution alone. An important first step is for clinical teachers to familiarize themselves with any conflict resolution (or problem-solving) models with which learners have experience, either from their educational programs or from their life experiences. When the curriculum does not stipulate the use of a model, clinical teachers need to be prepared for conflicts and have simple yet effective tools in place to help those involved in the conflicts to face them positively and constructively.

One such tool is a model that the American Management Association (n.d.) suggests. The model is an efficient five-step process for resolving conflict. First, identify the source of the conflict. Make sure that all parties have the chance to share their side of the story. Second, look beyond the incident. Explore perspectives of events and problems that might have triggered the incident. Third, request solutions. Ensure that each party identifies their idea of how the situation could be changed or resolved. Fourth, identify solutions that all parties can support. Point out the merits of various ideas, not only from each other's perspective, but also in terms of benefits to the organization. Fifth, reach agreement. Agree to an idea identified in the fourth step, possibly in the form of a written contract. Create a plan for what to do if problems arise in the future.

It is useful to introduce learners to whatever model will be used to resolve conflicts in their learning experiences before a distressing disagreement arises. Including an explanation of the model during orientation activities and commenting on how conflict is an expected and potentially positive aspect of clinical practice will normalize the experience. Just as collaborations that enhance emotional resilience, promote civility, and harness anxiety help health-care professionals to provide more compassionate care to patients/clients, so too when health-care professionals work toward resolving conflicting views patients/clients benefit once again (Ellis & Toney-Butler, 2019).

Nurturing an "attitude of gratitude" can prevent disagreements from escalating into distressing and emotionally depleting conflicts. Understanding others' perspectives is an important element of resolving conflict successfully. Cultivating and displaying positive emotions such as joy, optimism, and gratitude can help people to remain open to different ways of thinking and acting, even when they might not agree with these differences.

Research indicates that the positive emotion of gratitude is linked to lower levels of aggression and motivates people to express sensitivity to and concern for others (DeWall et al., 2012). Expressing gratitude can help people to feel less emotionally exhausted and cynical and more inclined to approach potential conflicts and problems proactively (Burke et al., 2009). A focus on positivity and gratitude shifts thinking away from negative emotions (Emmons & McCullough, 2003). In one health professions program, when faculty were introduced to gratitude interventions, they felt a deeper sense of appreciation for colleagues and more satisfaction with their jobs (Stegen & Wankier, 2018).

Gratitude can be construed as both an emotional response and a habit or coping response. In his work exploring gratitude, Robert Emmons (n.d.), the founding editor-in-chief of *The Journal of Positive Psychology*, encouraged people to view experiencing and expressing gratitude as a habit that can be developed and should be practised daily. He suggests establishing a daily practice of reminding ourselves of the good things that we enjoy, our personal attributes, and valued people in our lives and then recording them in a journal. When clinical teachers model an attitude of gratitude and invite students to do the same, they set a tone of reciprocal respect that enriches interactions and makes conflicts that emerge less onerous and emotionally damaging.

A Strategy to Try ▶ *Create a Personal Gratitude Collage*

At a regular time each clinical day, have students record one thing for which they are grateful. This could be something that they enjoy, a personal attribute, or a valued person in their lives. The record could be kept on a sticky note or other written material, or it could be kept online. Once students have a selection of separate gratitude records, perhaps at the midpoint of the learning experience, invite them to put them together into a gratitude collage. Create opportunities for students to share their collages with peers during group conferences. Make your own gratitude collage, refer to it often, and model an attitude of gratitude.

CONCLUSION

In this chapter, we discussed how maintaining resilience through positive collaborations can nurture feelings of fulfillment and passion. A career in the health professions, in which caring for others can be emotionally demanding, requires people to remain emotionally resilient. Connecting with others in meaningful ways can help those who provide care to others to receive needed emotional support themselves. Clinical teachers can cultivate successful collaborations with and among learners in everyday activities. Educators can intentionally provide safe spaces where learners are free to express their negative emotions as well as their positive emotions. They can encourage reflective practice, remain aware of the imbalance of power during supervision, and ensure that opportunities for connecting with like-minded others, such as fellow students, are available.

Importantly, during every interaction that clinical teachers engage in with learners, practitioners, patients/clients, and others in the clinical environment, they model the behaviour that they expect to see learners demonstrate. When clinical teachers use strategies that promote civility, harness anxiety, and resolve conflicts in their relationships with others, learners will assimilate these strategies into their own thinking.

In many instances, the personal connections with others sustain healthcare professionals during times when they feel emotionally depleted. Guiding learners toward establishing successful collaborations will strengthen their emotional well-being, increase their feelings of satisfaction at work, and ultimately help them to provide compassionate care to patients/clients.

REFERENCES

Aguilar, E. (2018). *Onward: Cultivating emotional resilience in educators.* Jossey-Bass.

Aiken, L., Sermeus, W., Van den Heede, K., Sloane, D. M., Busse, R., McKee, M., . . . Kutney-Lee, A. (2012). Patient safety, satisfaction, and quality of hospital care: Cross sectional surveys of nurses and patients in 12 countries in Europe and the United States. *British Medical Journal, 344,* Art. e1717. https://doi.org/10.1136/bmj.e1717

American Management Association. (n.d.) Five steps to conflict resolution [Blog]. https://www.amanet.org/articles/the-five-steps-to-conflict-resolution/

American Psychological Association. (2014). *The road to resilience.* American Psychological Association. http://www.apa.org/helpcenter/road-resilience.aspx

Andersen, T., & Watkins, K. (2018). The value of peer mentorship as an educational strategy in nursing. *Journal of Nursing Education, 57*(4), 217–224. https://doi.org/10.3928/01484834-20180322-05

Boyle, D. A. (2011). Countering compassion fatigue: A requisite nursing agenda. *Online Journal of Issues in Nursing, 16*(1), Manuscript 2. https://ojin.nursingworld.org/MainMenuCategories/ANAMarketplace/ANAPeriodicals/OJIN/TableofContents/Vol-16-2011/No1-Jan-2011/Countering-Compassion-Fatigue.html

Burke, R., Ng, E., & Fiksenbaum, L. (2009). Virtues, work satisfactions and psychological wellbeing among nurses. *International Journal of Workplace Health Management, 2*(3), 202–219. https://doi.org/10.1108/17538350910993403

Cheng, C., Bartram, T, Karimi, L., & Leggat, S. (2013). The role of team climate in the management of emotional labour: Implications for nurse retention. *Journal of Advanced Nursing, 69*(12), 2812–2824. https://doi.org/10.1111/jan.12202

Clark, C. M., & Carnosso, J. (2008). Civility: A concept analysis. *The Journal of Theory Construction & Testing, 12*(1), 11–15.

Clark, C. M., Farnsworth, J., & Landrum, R. E. (2009). Development and description of the incivility in nursing education (INE) survey. *The Journal of Theory Construction & Testing, 13*(1), 7–15.

Clark, C. M., & Springer, P. J. (2007). Incivility in nursing education: A descriptive study of definitions and prevalence. *Journal of Nursing Education, 46*(1), 7–14.

Colvin, J., & Ashman, M. (2010). Roles, risks and benefits of peer mentoring relationships in higher education. *Mentoring and Tutoring: Partnership in Learning, 18*(2), 121–134. https://doi.org/10.1080/13611261003678879

Craft, J., Schivinski, E., & Wright, A. (2020). The grim reality of nursing incivility. *Journal for Nurses in Professional Development, 36*(1), 41–43. https://doi.org/10.1097/NND.0000000000000599

Delgado, C., Roche, M., Fethney, J., & Foster, K. (2020). Workplace resilience and emotional labour of Australian mental health nurses: Results of a national survey. *International Journal of Mental Health Nursing, 29*(1), 35–46. https://doi.org/10.1111/inm.12598

Delgado, C., Upton, D., Ranse, K., Furness, T., & Foster, K. (2017). Nurses' resilience and the emotional labour of nursing work: An integrative review of empirical literature. *International Journal of Nursing Studies, 70*, 71–88. https://doi.org/ 10.1016/j.ijnurstu.2017.02.008

DeWall, C. N., Lambert, N. M., Pond, R. S., Kashdan, T. B., & Fincham, F. D. (2012). A grateful heart is a nonviolent heart: Cross-sectional, experience sampling, longitudinal, and experimental evidence. *Social Psychological and Personality Science, 3*(2), 232–240. https://doi.org/10.1177/1948550611416675

Eichbaum, Q. (2018). Collaboration and teamwork in the health professions: Rethinking the role of conflict. *Academic Medicine, 93*(4), 574–580. https://doi. org/10.1097/ACM.0000000000002015

Ellis, V., & Toney-Butler, T. (2019). *Conflict management.* StatPearls Publishing. https://www.ncbi.nlm.nih.gov/books/NBK470432/

Emmons, R. (n.d.). *Ten ways to become more grateful* [Website]. Greater Good Science Center at UC Berkeley. https://greatergood.berkeley.edu/article/item/ ten_ways_to_become_more_grateful1/

Emmons, R., & McCullough, M. (2003). Counting blessings versus burdens: An experiential investigation of gratitude and subjective well-being in daily life. *Journal of Personality and Social Psychology, 84*(2), 377–389. https://doi. org/10.1037/0022-3514.84.2.377

Eng, C., & Pai, H. (2015). Determinants of nursing competence of nursing students in Taiwan: The role of self-reflection and insight. *Nurse Education Today, 35*(3), 450–455.

Epstein, R. (1999). Mindful practice. *Journal of the American Medical Association, 282*(9), 833–839. https://doi.org/10.1001/jama.282.9.833

Foureur, M., Besley, K., Burton, G., Yu, N., & Crisp, J. (2013). Enhancing the resilience of nurses and midwives: Pilot of a mindfulness based program for increased health, sense of coherence and decreased depression, anxiety and stress. *Contemporary Nurse, 45*(1), 114–125. https://doi.org/10.5172/conu.2013.45.1.114

Fowler, M. (2015). Dealing with compassion fatigue. *New Jersey Education Association Review, 88*(7), 32–35.

Fredrickson, B. (2009). *Positivity: Groundbreaking research reveals how to embrace the hidden strength of positive emotions, overcome negativity, and thrive.* Crown.

Grant, L., & Kinman, G. (2014). Emotional resilience in the helping professions and how it can be enhanced. *Health and Social Care Education, 3*(1), 23–34. https:// doi.org/10.11120/hsce.2014.00040

Hartmann, S., Weiss, M., Newman, A., & Hoegl, M. (2020). Resilience in the workplace: A multilevel review and synthesis. *Applied Psychology, 69*, 913–959. https://doi.org/10.1111/apps.12191

Hochschild, A. R. (1983/2003). *The managed heart: Commercialization of human feeling.* University of California Press.

Hunsaker, S., Chen, H., Maughan, D., & Heaston, S. (2015). Factors that influence the development of compassion fatigue, burnout, and compassion satisfaction in emergency department nurses. *Journal of Nursing Scholarship, 47*(2), 186–194.

Irving, J., Dobkin, P., & Park, J. (2009). Cultivating mindfulness in health care professionals: A review of empirical studies of mindfulness-based stress reduction (MBSR). *Complementary Therapies in Clinical Practice, 15*, 61–66. https://doi.org/10.1016/j.ctcp.2009.01.002

Isenbarger, L., & Zembylas, M. (2006). The emotional labour of caring in teaching. *Teaching and Teacher Education, 2*, 120–134.

Kinman, G., & Leggetter, S. (2016). Emotional labour and wellbeing: What protects nurses? *Healthcare, 4*(4), 89. https://doi.org/10.3390/healthcare4040089

Krop, J. (2013). Caring without tiring. *Education Canada, 53*(2), Article 4.

Layne, D., Nemeth, L., Mueller, M., & Mart, M. (2019). Negative behaviors among healthcare professionals: Relationship with patient safety culture. *Healthcare, 7*(1), 23. https://doi.org/10.3390/healthcare7010023

Maslach, C., Jackson, S., & Leiter, M. (1996). *The Maslach burnout inventory* (3rd ed.). Consulting Psychologists Press.

McAllister, M., & McKinnon, J. (2009). The importance of teaching and learning resilience in the health disciplines: A critical literature review. *Nurse Education Today, 29*, 371–379. https://doi.org/10.1016/j.nedt.2008.10.011

McCann, C. M., Beddoe, E., McCormick, K., Huggard, P., Kedge, S., Adamson, C., & Huggard, J. (2013). Resilience in the health professions: A review of recent literature. *International Journal of Wellbeing, 3*(1), 60–81. https://doi.org/10.5502/ijw.v3i1.4

Melincavage, S. M. (2011). Student nurses' experiences of anxiety in the clinical setting. *Nurse Education Today, 31*(8), 785–789.

Melo, K., Williams, B., & Ross, C. (2010). The impact of nursing curricula on clinical practice anxiety. *Nurse Education Today, 30*, 773–778.

Melrose, S., Park, C., & Perry, B. (2020). *Centring human connections in the education of health professionals.* Athabasca University Press.

Milesky, J., Baptiste, D., Foronda, C., Dupler, A., & Belcher, A. (2015). Promoting a culture of civility in nursing education and practice. *Journal of Nursing Education and Practice, 5*(8), 90–94. https://doi.org/10.5430/jnep.v5n8p90

Oyeleye, O., Hanson, P., O'Connor, N., & Dunn, D. (2013). Relationship of workplace incivility, stress, and burnout on nurses' turnover intentions and psychological empowerment. *Journal of Nursing Administration, 43*(10), 536–542.

Palmer, p. (2007). *The courage to teach: Exploring the inner landscape of a teacher's life.* Jossey-Bass.

Pattani, R., Ginsburg, S., Mascarenhas Johnson, A., Moore, J. E., Jassemi, S., & Straus, S. E. (2018). Organizational factors contributing to incivility at an academic medical center and systems-based solutions: A qualitative study. *Academic Medicine: Journal of the Association of American Medical Colleges, 93*(10), 1569–1575. https://doi.org/10.1097/ACM.0000000000002310

Penconek, T. (2014). *Beware of uncharitable speech: Perceptions of newly graduated nurses regarding their experiences of academic incivility between and among nursing students in undergraduate nursing education* (Unpublished master's thesis). Athabasca University, Athabasca, AB.

Penconek, T. (2020). Theoretical approaches to studying incivility in nursing education. *International Journal of Nursing Education Scholarship, 17*(1), Art. 20190060. https://doi.org/10.1515/ijnes-2019-0060

Pipe, T., Buchda, V., Lauder, S., Hudak, B., Hulvey, L., Karns, K & Pendergast, D. (2012). Building personal resources of resilience and agility in the healthcare workplace. *Stress and Health: Journal of the International Society for the Investigation of Stress, 28*(1), 11-22. https://doi.org/ 10.1002/smi.1396

Porath, C., & Pearson, C. (2013). The price of incivility. *Harvard Business Review, 91*(1–2) 114–121, 146.

Pronovost, P., & Vohr, E. (2010). *Safe patients, smart hospitals.* Hudson Street Press.

Rakesh, G., Pier, K., & Costales, T. (2017). A call for action: Cultivating resilience in healthcare providers. *The American Journal of Psychiatry Residents' Journal, 12*(4), 3–5. https://doi.org/10.1176/appi.ajp-rj.2017.120402

Rees, C., Breen, L., Cusack, L., & Hegney, D. (2015). Understanding individual resilience in the workplace: The international collaboration of workforce resilience model. *Frontiers in Psychology, 6,* Article 73. https://doi.org/10.3389/fpsyg.2015.00073

Reid, D. (2013). Teaching mindfulness to occupational therapy students: Pilot evaluation of an online curriculum. *Canadian Journal of Occupational Therapy, 80*(1), 42–48. https://doi.org/10.1177/0008417413475598

Robertson, J. E. (2012). Can't we all just get along? A primer on student incivility in nursing education. *Nursing Education Perspectives, 33*(1), 21–26.

Ruiz-Martin, C., Lopez-Paredes, A., & Wainer, G. (2018). What we know and do not know about organizational resilience. *International Journal of Production Management and Engineering, 6*(1), 11–28. https://doi.org/10.4995/ijpme.2018.7898

Shapiro, S. (2009). The integration of mindfulness and psychology. *Journal of Clinical Psychology, 65*(6), 555–560. https://doi.org/10.1002/jclp.20602

Showalter, S. (2010). Compassion fatigue: What is it? Why does it matter? *American Journal of Hospice & Palliative Medicine, 27*(4), 239–242.

Sprengel, A. D., & Job, L. (2004). Reducing student anxiety by using clinical peer mentoring with beginning nursing students. *Nurse Educator, 29*(6), 246–250.

Stacey, G., Aubeeluck, A., Cook, G., & Dutta, S. (2017). A case study exploring the experience of resilience-based clinical supervision and its influence on care towards self and others among student nurses. *International Practice Development Journal, 7*(2), Article 5. https://doi.org/10.19043/ipdj.72.005

Stacey, G., & Cook, G. (2019). A scoping review exploring how the conceptualization of resilience in nursing influences interventions aimed at increasing resilience. *International Practice Development Journal, 9*(1), Article 9. https://doi.org/10.19043/ipdj.91.009

Stegen, A., & Wankier, J. (2018). Generating gratitude in the workplace to improve faculty job satisfaction. *Journal of Nursing Education, 57*(6), 375–378.

Stephens, T. (2013). Nursing student resilience: A concept clarification. *Nursing Forum, 48*(2), 125–133. https://doi.org/10.1111/nuf.12015

Thomas, C., Bantz, D. & McIntosh, C. (2019). Nurse faculty burnout and strategies to avoid it. *Teaching and Learning in Nursing, 14*, 111–116. https://doi.org/10.1016/j.teln.2018.12.005

Tugade, M. M., Fredrickson, B. L., & Barrett, L. F. (2004). Psychological resilience and positive emotional granularity: Examining the benefits of positive emotions on coping and health. *Journal of Personality, 72*(6), 1161–1190. https://doi.org/10.1111/j.1467-6494.2004.00294.x

Turner, K., & McCarthy, V. (2016). Stress and anxiety among nursing students: A review of intervention strategies in literature between 2009 and 2015. *Nurse Education in Practice, 22*, 21–29.

World Health Organization. (2018). Burn-out. In Chapter 24, Factors influencing health status or contact with health services. *International statistical classification of diseases and related health problems* (11th revision). https://icd.who.int/browse11/l-m/en

Zhu, Z., Xing, W., Lizarondo, L., Guo, M., & Hu, Y. (2019). Nursing students' experiences with faculty incivility in the clinical education context: A qualitative systematic review and meta-synthesis. *BMJ Open, 9*(2), Art. e024383. https://doi.org/10.1136/bmjopen-2018-024383

5

Professional Socialization of Health-Care Professionals

Thought flows in terms of stories—stories about events, stories about people, and stories about intentions and achievements. The best teachers are the best storytellers. We learn in the form of stories.

FRANK SMITH (1992, P. 62)

Today's clinical learning environments can seem to be overwhelming. Students in the health-care professions face a complex and stressful transition from learners to competent practitioners. How do students make the transition from struggling beginners to fully functioning professionals? The transition occurs in part during pre-service education. However, educating health-care professionals is more than teaching them to deliver a series of skills successfully. Students also need to be guided in developing professional values and identities through socialization.

Socialization for health-care professionals can have two aspects. *Organizational socialization* is fitting into the structure of the organization, maintaining relationships with colleagues, learning the organizational culture, and learning the formal and informal rules of the practice environment. *Professional socialization* is internalization of a set of values and the culture of the profession (Zarshenas et el., 2014). Furthermore, professional socialization is the process by which students develop a sense of themselves as members of a profession, internalize the values of their profession, and exhibit these values through their behaviour (Gaberson et al., 2014; Nordstrom et al., 2018; Weidman et al., 2001). The focus of this chapter is the professional socialization of learners in health-care professions. We present a variety of creative strategies that clinical teachers can incorporate into group or conference activities with students.

Professional socialization involves guiding learners to make personal commitments to their chosen profession. This commitment leads to actions and attitudes that are described by Black (2013, p. 118) as "thinking like a nurse" or another health-care professional. A professional identity evolves from effective professional socialization (MacLellan et al., 2011; Mooney, 2007), and professional socialization is a foundation of effective practice (Perry, 2009a).

Here we assume that professional socialization is a desirable outcome. Although many authors discuss socialization exclusively as a positive goal for educators, others focus on the potentially negative effects of socialization, such as group-think and undermining of diversity. Benner et al. (2010, p. 86) choose to use the term "formation" to represent the positive effects of workplace learning and to consider socialization as something that can exert positive or negative influence. We consider professional socialization an important learning outcome for students and a task for health-care educators. In this chapter, we provide a primer on professional socialization and then discuss how storytelling and role modelling contribute to professional socialization.

A PRIMER ON PROFESSIONAL SOCIALIZATION

Through professional socialization processes, educators support learners as they gradually develop a sense of belonging to specific professional groups. Professional socialization occurs through a combination of professional education and clinical experience (Beck, 2014). In a study of Japanese nursing students, Condon & Sharts-Hopko (2010) found that professional socialization is multidimensional and includes influences from classroom experience, clinical practice, and extracurricular elements. Zarshenas et al. (2014) explored factors that affect professional socialization of nursing students and discovered that a sense of belonging and professional identity underlies successful professional socialization. More specifically, this sense of belonging develops through educational experiences and tacit knowledge; acquiring professional identity evolves in part from internal motivation and role modelling.

Professional socialization is considered a process that begins on day one of formal education programs and continues as learners graduate and enter the workforce. Peers, instructors, preceptors, mentors, and patients/clients and their families can all be socializing agents (Chitty & Black, 2011). Black (2013) emphasizes that socialization occurs through a combination of formal and informal processes (e.g., unplanned observations). She notes that, to be most effective, formal socialization in educational programs should occur through a deliberate, systematic, block-building process. Socialization occurs in part in the clinical setting, in which learning outcomes are often achieved through observation of other practitioners who demonstrate a commitment to professional values. The clinical setting is also where learners are held accountable for their actions and the outcomes of their interventions are apparent (Gaberson et al., 2014).

Studies with social work students reveal how difficult it can be to measure values and attitudes accurately (Barretti, 2004) and to understand how changes actually occur (Valutis et al., 2012; Weiss et al., 2004). In physical therapy, the professional socialization process is highly influenced by interactions with peers and faculty (Teschendorf & Nemshick, 2001). For student athletic trainers, professional socialization is effected by legitimation from socializing agents, such as patients and clinical instructors (Klossner, 2008), and by communication with practitioners (Mensch et al., 2005).

Educators who actively guide learners toward professional socialization are generally agreed to be important. Although educators might set out to assist learners in graduating fully socialized for their professions, many report feeling unprepared to fulfill this role (Clark & Holmes, 2007; O'Shea & Kelly, 2007). Furthermore, though new graduates have the competencies for licensure, concern remains about their socialization to professional practice (Gaberson et al., 2014). Feng and Tsai (2012) conclude that new graduates are often stressed when organizational and professional values clash. More specifically, they find that the organizational value of task-oriented nursing clashes with the professional value of patient-oriented nursing, resulting in distress for neophyte nurses. Clinical educators must therefore deliberately include strategies to help learners become socialized to their professions. Understanding professional identity and values provides a foundation that can help to develop these deliberate strategies.

Professional identity is a form of social identity by which members of a profession categorize and differentiate themselves from other professions (Schein, 1978). Professional identity is categorized by Wackerhausen (2009) as macro (status, privileges, duties, and self-image of the profession) and micro (tacit behavioural norms of the profession enacted by individuals). According to Enns (2014), nursing professional identity is born from values and encompasses both the individual's sense of self as a nurse and the image of a nurse that the person projects to others. Professional socialization, in part through formal education, means that individuals are likely to identify strongly with their own professional group (Coyle et al., 2011).

Professional values, one essential element of professional socialization, are key to success as a practitioner since they provide a foundation for behaviour (Chitty & Black, 2011). Professional values are the *blueprint for action* for exemplary care providers (Perry, 2009a).

Values are defined by Schwartz (1994, p. 21) as "guiding principles in the life of a person that motivate action, function as standards for judging and justifying action, and that are acquired both through socialization and through the unique learning experiences." Some research indicates that existing values can influence career choice. For example, Adams et al. (2006) propose that nursing students are guided in their career choice in part because their personal values align with those of the profession. In other words, students might begin their training programs with certain values in place that are desired by the profession. Although the values favoured by dissimilar professions can vary, Thorpe and Loo (2003) discovered that the values of altruism (a desire to help others) and personal development (a desire to develop as a person) influence the choice of nursing as a career. Fagermoen (1997, p. 439), one of the early researchers who linked values to certain professions, concluded that common core nursing values include dignity, personhood, being a fellow human, reciprocal trust, and personalization of care. Because of the likely link between values and professional identity, Adams et al. (2006) conclude that new nursing students have some professional identity prior to professional socialization (see figure 1).

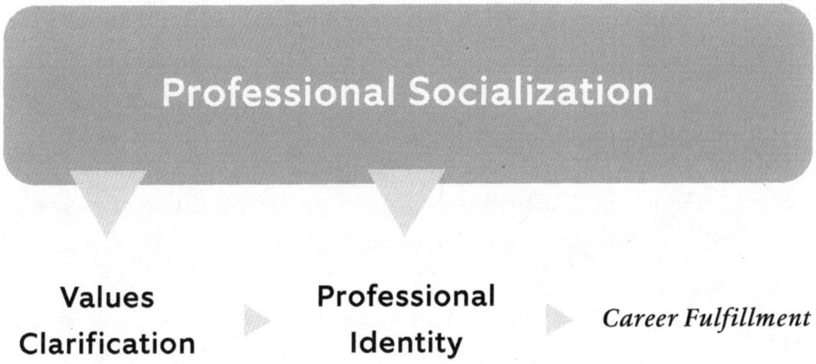

Professional Socialization

Values Clarification ▷ Professional Identity ▷ *Career Fulfillment*

Figure 1. The association among professional socialization, values clarification, professional identity, and career fulfillment.

A Strategy to Try ▷ *Minute at the Movies*

To encourage learners to reflect on their values and beliefs, you can use examples of human interaction from movies or other media as triggers for new learner insights. For this group or conference activity, provide students with brief clips from inspiring movies related to their real-time clinical situations. For example, to trigger reflection and discussion related to palliative care and the meaning of life and death, you could show the trailer from *A Fault in Our Stars* or *Wit* at a post-practicum conference.

Students watch the clip and share their observations in response to a specific reflection question that you provide. In this example, the reflection question could be as simple as "What did this movie teach you about dying?" Often students bring in their own examples from other movies or television shows that they find relevant, furthering the breadth and depth of the discussion.

One foundation of providing competent health care might be professional socialization that develops professional identity and values. Bernard et al. (2003, p. 64) state that values are the foundation of our attitudes and beliefs that "encapsulate the aspirations of individuals and societies and encompass deeply engrained standards that determine future directions and justify past actions." Thus, professionals determine priorities, weigh options, and choose actions based on values (Bardi et al., 2009).

In linking professional identity and values, Fagermoen (1997, p. 436) concludes that "values are inherent in developing and sustaining professional identity and are expressed in . . . actions in relation to others." Furthermore, applying core values in professional practice increases work satisfaction, which continues the cycle of value enactment (Perry, 2009a). More specifically, nurses who perceive that they provide high-quality care and make strong connections with their patients are usually very satisfied with their career choice (Perry, 2005).

A Strategy to Try ▶ *The Health Professional I Would Like to Be*

Invite students to describe the characteristics or qualities of a health-care professional whom they know or to imagine a perfect health-care professional in their field. Discuss the common qualities and characteristics of the professionals whom they aspire to be like. Ask them to reflect on their current images of themselves as health-care professionals and to compare these images with their ideal images. Have them identify two areas that they would like to focus on for improvement.

STORYTELLING

Clinical educators are positioned to cultivate professional identity and selected values, leading to effective professional socialization of health-care learners. The clinical setting is rich in opportunities for educators to use learning activities and teaching strategies that achieve what are often learning outcomes from the affective domain. Methods of teaching psychomotor skills and cognitive knowledge are often more straightforward. Effective clinical educators take the challenge to reach learners on emotional and attitudinal levels. Storytelling is an effective strategy that invites students to make links among the professionals whom they hope to be, the values that they hold, and the career fulfillment that they desire.

Using arts-based teaching strategies helps students to make an emotional connection to their learning, caters to a variety of learning styles, and increases student achievement (Perry & Edwards, 2015). Arts-based approaches can stimulate creative, critical, and analytical teaching about clinical situations. Telling stories is a teaching approach rooted in the arts. It can have positive effects on teacher-learner and learner-learner rapport, interaction, and community building. Art moves individuals to look at broader concepts and ideas, encouraging them to look at multiple facets and dimensions. Learners are encouraged to move away from breaking knowledge into discrete elements for analytical assessment and from looking at learning as a checklist or assembly line of tasks. Since professional socialization is more non-concrete, it requires multilayered and complex strategies that inspire thinking broadly, deeply, and holistically.

Clinical instructors can use relevant stories about patients to trigger transformative learning. Stories can come from many sources, including the instructor's personal repertoire of clinical experiences, published clinical stories, or students themselves. To be the most effective, storytelling should be a deliberate and guided learning activity. Stories need to be carefully selected for their relevance to the clinical situation, learners' level, and desired value or attitude lessons. After sharing the story (either verbally or in written form), the instructor should be prepared to lead a discussion that guides learners to express their reflections and evaluate their conclusions. A summation of the learning experience will help learners to clarify and reinforce take-away concepts and ideas.

EMOTIONAL CONNECTIONS

The following is an example of a story that can create emotional connections with learning. This story can be used by nursing instructors in a post-clinical face-to-face conference or an online discussion forum after a shift on a medical unit.

> A year or so ago, I was working nights. My patient became increasingly restless and agitated. He had a progressive dementia and he was more disturbed than any patient I had cared for in my 25 years or more of nursing. That night, he required two-to-one nursing care.
>
> Around 0300 hours the other nurse I was working with observed that, in spite of his verbal lashing out, he had never once cursed. She remarked that he must not have "bad" words in his normal vocabulary because usually what is in a mind comes out in confusion. The night wore on with our patient experiencing agitation, yelling and extreme restlessness. He would bite his own hands and arms and grab on to anything near him. We began to wonder if we could ever help him rest. I remember feeling helpless and hopeless.
>
> Then I heard him repeat a series of words in a garbled fashion and recognized the words of an old hymn. I began to sing the hymn and immediately he became quiet. The change was instantaneous and profound. The other nurse was able to leave for a break while I sat beside him singing every hymn I could remember.
>
> As long as the hymns were sung, the patient rested. (The nurse added a side note saying that it was a good thing she was a pk—a preacher's kid—and because of this, she knew a lot of hymns). We later found out that the man had been a lay pastor, and perhaps this explained his reaction to my music.
>
> I loved being his nurse because none of the usual text-book interventions worked. He required flexible, creative nurses who were not afraid to try the unconventional and who were willing to keep trying until we could find a way to connect with him and his needs. Large doses of artificial sedation made no difference. Somewhere in the deepest levels of this man's mind, our presence through music and just being near touched him. It was a profound night because all my years of training and education came down to the simple singing of a song. (Perry, 2009a, p. 210)

A storytelling strategy in clinical teaching can stimulate learners to interact with their colleagues in sharing their insights and comparing their analyses. Connectedness, interrelatedness, and integration can be an outcome when arts are the foundation of teaching strategies (Eccles & Elster, 2005). As Clarke and Widdicombe (2002, p. 45) conclude, the arts as a component of teaching strategies engage students totally, "not just with pen and pencil, but also with imagination."

A Strategy to Try ▶ *Sharing an Inspirational Story*
Share an inspirational story with your students. Include how the story reflects your own journey toward professional identity, your own values, and how it contributed to career fulfillment.

A Strategy to Try ▶ *The Patient I Will Always Remember*
This learning activity is also rooted in the arts and in storytelling but takes a slightly different approach. The exercise requires instructors to be reflective and willing to be emotionally vulnerable to learners. You can recall and share with learners the story of a person whom you cared for in clinical practice. Your story can be shared orally or in writing and should be accompanied by guided reflection and discussion questions. The clinical post-conference (either face-to-face or in an online discussion forum) is an appropriate setting for this learning activity. The success of this learning activity depends heavily on careful selection of the patient example to make it appropriate to the learners and to the clinical setting. The following is an example of a story told by an instructor to a group of nursing students during a public health clinical rotation.

> This patient I remember often was a street person. She had lived a hard life. It was beyond anything I had ever experienced. Her hard life was paralleled by her equally hard death. When she did come in to clinic, she was dirty, dishevelled, often carrying insects in her backpack and on her frail body. Other staff freaked out when she came in, afraid of bed bugs and lice and afraid of her because her life script was so different from theirs. She actually didn't have a home, so home care was not an option. She didn't have a home, but

she did have a cellphone, and when I would call to check on her pain level or some other issue and I would ask "Where are you?" she would answer matter-of-factly "On my bench." She had taken ownership of a park bench, and this was her "home."

Although her life was far different from mine, there was something that drew me to her. I came to know her well over her years of treatment, and I always tried to make time to hear at least one of her street stories. I listened to her, to her words, but also to the embedded messages and cries for help. I would like to be able to say I was able to whisk her into a clean hospice room and fix all her social and emotional issues, but this wasn't to be. In the end, she died in her own world, but I hope she knew at least one other person cared about her.

TRANSFORMATIONS

Storytelling can create transformations in the way that learners think about and view the world. Mezirow (1981) defines transformational learning as critically reflecting on our assumptions and beliefs, then intentionally creating a new view of the world. He labels this "perspective transformation." O'Sullivan (1999) emphasizes that transformative learning involves a deep shift in consciousness that changes a person's view of her or his place in the world. Introducing educational approaches that challenge learners consciously to examine their unrecognized underlying views and assumptions can transform their views of the world. Learning approaches that challenge students to question what they believe to be true, and ultimately to interpret information more critically, can be transformative (Melrose et al., 2013).

Research supports the potential influence of transformational learning strategies on the development of values. Williams et al. (2012) describe transformational learning approaches that enhance the development of values among nursing students. Such approaches must be based on active, realistic experiences that engage students in self-directed inquiry and critical thinking. More specifically, Williams et al. report that an effective strategy for professional socialization is to have students work in small peer groups to discuss real practice scenarios. Those exposed to this learning strategy are self-directed learners and advocates for patients and their profession upon graduation.

In the clinical situation, the strategy of practice scenarios used by Williams et al. (2012) could become real scenarios within a storytelling teaching approach rather than fictitious cases. Opportunity for students to share their clinical experiences with one another and facilitated deconstruction and discussion of these scenarios in small groups or conferences, offer the potential for transformational learning. How can clinical instructors skilfully guide these discussions to optimize this potential? Before attitudinal shifts can occur, learners need to reflect critically on assumptions that they believe are true. Challenging these assumptions, at both a cognitive level and an emotional level, can be difficult, and the process of reflection is unlikely to be spontaneous. Instead, instructors must provide learners with opportunities to question their views on specific ideas or issues. Activities with no right or wrong interpretations can stimulate critical reflection.

A Strategy to Try ▶ *Which Patient Would I Choose?*
This strategy is one way that you can guide students in uncovering their assumptions about patients' race, gender, sexual orientation, socio-economic status, et cetera. In this learning activity, hold a group debriefing session after a clinical practice shift. Ensure a private setting where students can speak openly about their experiences. Have each student report briefly on a person whom he or she cared for during the shift, ensuring that the student includes the patient's biographical details as well as health status updates. Next ask learners to select the two patients, from those described by their peers, whom they would choose to care for if they had the option to select. The students should also identify the two patients whom they would choose not to care for. Then ask learners to consider why they made their choices and record any common themes that they observe in their own choices. After working on their choices individually, students should share their choices of patients and their reasons for choosing them. The goal of this activity is to help students examine their deeply held values, biases, and attitudes. Value awareness can be an initial step in value transformation and professional identity development.

GIVING VOICE WITH A PHOTO

Mezirow (1981) emphasizes the importance of providing challenges within educational processes. Teachers who challenge learners provide them with opportunities to question commonly accepted values and to reflect critically on points of view that are different from their own. Using selected photographs as an approach to storytelling can challenge learners. The photo selected must be relevant to the clinical setting and should be chosen to challenge specific values, assumptions, and attitudes that students might hold. The image can be circulated during a group learning activity, such as a post-clinical conference, to focus students' attention and initiate discussion of reflection questions provided by the instructor. As an alternative, students can be asked to provide images that challenge their attitudes and values and make them consider alternative views. These student-generated images can also be shared and discussed as a group.

Many open educational sources offer images that can be used for educational purposes. For example, Flickr is Creative Commons licensed, and images can be downloaded and printed for educational purposes.

ROLE MODELLING

Merton (1949/1957/1968) introduced role modelling as the process by which medical students in his study compared themselves with a reference group. Bandura's (1963) social learning theory furthered our understanding of how imitation and observation of others contributes to human learning. Modelling and Role Modelling (MRM) theory, developed by Erickson, Tomlin, and Swain (1983/2010), proposes that, when learners observe models, they perceive another person's point of view, values, and framework. The results are learner growth and improvement.

Role models influence students' values and professional identity development, and experiences with role models can facilitate transformational learning. In a study of effective role modelling in nursing education, Mokhtari Nouri et al. (2014) conclude that educators need to pay attention to personal and environmental factors. These investigators also conclude that observational learning through role modelling is especially important in clinical settings. In such settings, instructors both teach skills and demonstrate values and attitudes as learners come to reflect what they see and hear.

Helping learners to attain learning outcomes from the affective domain is challenging, but role modelling is one strategy to support attitudinal and emotional growth (Perry, 2009b). Cultivating attitudes such as compassion and caring is complex, so reaching these learning outcomes can create emotional challenges for students and instructors (Curtis, 2014). Modelling of compassionate practice by a skilled clinical instructor or preceptor is one strategy for furthering the adoption of a professional attitude and identity by health-care learners.

The following is an example of an exemplary nurse as a role model, recorded in field notes by Perry (2009a). The role model taught the nursing intervention of touch to establish connection with a patient, a skill that is challenging to teach in any way but through modelling.

> She often sits on the bed next to her patients, or she stands very close to their chairs. This physical closeness seems to create an air of familiarity. It makes their relationship close very quickly. It was by touching, by holding her patient's hand, laying a cold cloth on her forehead, and rubbing her sore back, that the nurse communicated that she cared. All that she did with touch said how much she wanted to help. (Perry, 2009a, p. 81)

Do slowly, think aloud. Model teachers facilitate emotional growth in learners by demonstrating effective interactions and interventions. Clinical educators need to embrace the reality that everything learners see their instructors do or hear them say (or not say) might influence the socialization and eventual success of graduates. This is a heavy responsibility, but it is the reality of accepting the role of clinical instructor. Instructors who choose to maximize the potential positive effects of their role modelling might deliberately slow down their actions and interventions to allow learners time to observe fully and absorb what is happening. When appropriate role models speak aloud their rationales for selected actions and interventions, they maximize the teaching potential of a situation.

The following example of a role model (exemplary nurse) demonstrates nursing interventions in such a manner.

> Her patient tonight can't talk. Each breath is a struggle. He is so afraid that the next breath just won't be there. In his eyes I see an unmistakable look of panic. A laryngeal cancer and tracheostomy

have taken his vocal cords and a tonsillar tumour has impaired his hearing. How can she let him know that she is there, that she cares? She works slowly. She doesn't say a word. As she strokes his hair, her eyes tell him what he so desperately wants to hear: that she is with him, that she will stay, that she will watch over him. Gradually, silently, he drifts off to sleep. When we return to the med room she tells me her beliefs about the importance of the nursing intervention of silence and touch in communicating caring. (Perry, 2009a, p. 60)

Admit it when you make a mistake. No one is perfect, including clinical educators. The educator might be less than perfectly prepared mentally, physically, or intellectually to model exemplary care on some days. Learners can observe errors in judgment, responses that are less than therapeutic, or rushed interventions. Reflective educators will be aware of possible negative modelling and openly discuss their reflections with learners. Together the instructor and students should analyze the situation and develop more optimal approaches to be used in subsequent patient care situations.

Cultivate opportunities to role-model. Since role modelling is a powerful teaching tool for health-care learners, clinical instructors should seek opportunities to model specific professional values and attitudes that they want to cultivate in students. Clearly articulating these desired values and attitudes in learning outcomes can highlight points that educators will focus on modelling. For example, if students are to develop strategies for respectful communication, then role models should prepare themselves to demonstrate this and watch for opportunities to have students observe them. Follow-up with learners is important to be sure that the role modelling is effective and that students internalize the desired learning.

Use humour appropriately. Humour is seeing what is funny in everyday encounters and maintaining a lighthearted attitude (when appropriate) in potentially difficult situations (Perry, 2009b). Curtis (2014) notes that learners value an appropriate sense of humour in role models and find that it facilitates their learning. Role models who use humour effectively and appropriately help students to manage their feelings of vulnerability and maintain their emotional well-being in challenging clinical situations.

Consider using social media. Students can receive role modelling from a variety of sources. Clinical teachers are an obvious source of modelling, but other health-care professionals in the clinical environment often model positively or negatively. In negative situations, instructors need to provide learners with opportunities to discuss and interpret what they observe. Social media such as Twitter can also provide a type of modelling for learners. In one example, students sought to develop leadership skills for the clinical setting. They were invited to follow the Twitter feed of a well-known leader in their profession and to extract leadership lessons from what they read. Students were asked to write a paper translating these leadership lessons into effective leadership approaches in the clinical setting. The activity encouraged learners to seek role models from a variety of sources and to participate in higher-order learning through analysis and evaluation. Learners are motivated to engage in this activity in part because of its novelty and in part because it uses a medium with which they are familiar and comfortable.

CONCLUSION

Fully educating health-care professionals includes helping them to become socialized to their professions. Clinical educators have an important opportunity and responsibility to guide learners in developing professional values and identities as steps in the process of professional socialization. Health-care students can bring deeply seated and well-established beliefs and assumptions to their learning. Cultivating selected values and attitudes can be a challenge for educators. Formation and transformation are possible in part through approaches such as storytelling and role modelling. Clinical educators can utilize creative teaching approaches akin to transformational learning pedagogy to facilitate professional socialization in learners.

REFERENCES

Adams, K., Hean, S., Sturgis, P., & Macleod-Clark, J. (2006). Investigating the factors influencing professional identity of first-year health and social care students. *Learning in Health and Social Care, 5*(2), 55–68. https://doi.org/10.1111/j.1473-6861.2006.00119.x

Bandura, A. (1963). *Social learning and personality development.* Holt, Rinehart, and Winston.

Bardi, A., Lee, J. A., Hofmann-Towfigh, N., & Soutar, G. (2009). The structure of intraindividual value change. *Journal of Personality and Social Psychology, 97*(5), 913–929. https://doi.org/10.1037/a0016617

Barretti, M. (2004). What do we know about the professional socialization of our students? *Journal of Social Work Education, 40*(2), 255–283.

Beck, J. W. (2014). Deconstructing student perceptions of incivility in nursing education. *Journal of Management Education, 38*(2), 160–191. https://doi.org/10.1177/1052562913488112

Benner, P., Sutphen, M., Leonard, V., & Day, L. (2010). *Educating nurses: A call for transformation.* Jossey-Bass.

Bernard, M., Maio, G., & Olson, J. (2003). The vulnerability of values to attack: Inoculation of values and value-relevant attitudes. *Personality and Social Psychology Bulletin, 29,* 63–75.

Black, B. p. (2013). *Professional nursing: Concepts and challenges* (7th ed.). Saunders Elsevier.

Chitty, K. K., & Black, B. p. (2011). *Becoming a nurse: Professional nursing: Concepts and challenges* (6th ed.). Saunders Elsevier.

Clark, T., & Holmes, S. (2007). Fit for practice? An exploration of the development of new qualified nurses using focus groups. *International Journal of Nursing Studies, 44,* 1210–1220.

Clarke, P., & Widdicombe, J. (2002). Making a new connection: Inner-city arts training program. *Education Canada, 42*(2), 44–45.

Condon, E., & Sharts-Hopko, N. (2010). Socialization of Japanese nursing students. *Nursing Education Perspectives, 31,* 167–170.

Coyle, J., Higgs, J., McAllister, L., & Whiteford, G. (2011). What is an interprofessional health care team anyway? In S. Kitto, J. Chesters, J. Thistelthwaite, & S. Reeves (Eds.), *Sociology of interprofessional health care practice: Critical reflections and concrete solutions* (pp. 39–53). Nova Science.

Curtis, K. (2014). Learning the requirements for compassionate practice: Student vulnerability and courage. *Nursing Ethics, 21*(2), 210–223. https://doi.org/10.1177/0969733013478307

Eccles, K., & Elster, A. (2005). Learning through the arts: A new school of thought? *Education Canada, 45*(3), 45–48.

Enns, B. (2014). *Finding my own way: Nursing identity development from layperson to new BN graduate* (Unpublished master's thesis). Athabasca University, Athabasca, AB. https://dt.athabascau.ca/jspui/bitstream/10791/37/5/Enns_Finding_my_own_way.pdf

Erickson, H., Tomlin, E., & Swain, M. (1983/2010). *Modeling and role-modeling: A theory and paradigm for nursing.* Prentice-Hall.

Fagermoen, M. S. (1997). Professional identity: Values embedded in meaningful nursing practice. *Journal of Advanced Nursing, 25*(3), 434–441. https://doi.org/ 10.1046/j.1365-2648.1997.1997025434.x

Feng, R., & Tsai, Y. (2012). Socialisation of new graduate nurses to practising nurses. *Journal of Clinical Nursing, 21*(13–14), 2064–2071. https://doi.org/10.1111/ j.1365-2702.2011.03992.x

Gaberson, K. B., Oermann, M. H., & Shellenbarger, T. (2014). *Clinical teaching strategies in nursing* (4th ed.). Springer.

Klossner, J. (2008). The role of legitimation in the professional socialization of second-year undergraduate athletic training students. *Journal of Athletic Training, 43*(4), 379–385.

MacLellan, D., Lordly, D., & Gingras, J. (2011). Professional socialization in dietetics: A review of the literature. *Canadian Journal of Dietetic Practice and Research, 72*(1), 37–42.

Melrose, S., Park, C., & Perry, B. (2013). *Teaching health professionals online.* Athabasca University Press. https://doi.org/10.15215/aupress/9781927356654.01

Mensch, J., Crews, C., & Mitchell, M. (2005). Competing perspectives during organizational socialization on the role of certified athletic trainers in high school settings. *Journal of Athletic Training, 40*(4), 333–340.

Merton, R. K. (1949/1957/1968). *Social theory and social structure.* Free Press.

Mezirow, J. (1981). A critical theory of adult learning and education. *Adult Education Quarterly, 32*, 3–23.

Mokhtari Nouri, J., Ebadi, A., Alhani, F., & Rejeh, N. (2014). Experiences of role model instructors and nursing students about facilitator factors of role-modeling process: A qualitative research. *Iranian Journal of Nursing & Midwifery Research, 19*(3), 248–254.

Mooney, M. (2007). Professional socialization: The key to survival as a newly qualified nurse. *International Journal of Nursing Practice, 13*, 75–80.

Nordstrom, P., Currie, G., & Meyer, S. (2018). Becoming a nurse: Student experience of transformation and professional identity. *Quality Advancement in Nursing Education, 4*(2), Art. 4. https://doi.org/10.17483/2368-6669.115

O'Shea, M., & Kelly, B. (2007). The lived experiences of newly qualified nurses on clinical placement during the first six months following registration in the Republic of Ireland. *Journal of Clinical Nursing, 16*, 1534–1542.

O'Sullivan, E. (1999). *Transformative learning: Educational vision for the twenty-first century.* University of Toronto Press. http://wiki.sugarlabs.org/images/8/ 8a/O%27Sullivan19xxch8.pdf

Perry, B. (2005). Core values brought to life through stories. *Nursing Standard, 20*(7), 41–48.

Perry, B. (2009a). *More moments in time: Images of exemplary nursing.* Athabasca University Press.

Perry, B. (2009b). Role modeling excellence in clinical nursing practice. *Nurse Education Practice, 9,* 36–44.

Perry, B., & Edwards, M. (2015). Arts-based technologies create community in online courses. In G. Veletsianos (Ed.), *Emerging technologies in distance education* (2nd ed., 129–152). Athabasca University Press.

Schein, E. H. (1978). *Career dynamics: Matching individual and organisational needs.* Addison-Wesley.

Schwartz, S. H. (1994). Are there universal aspects in the content and structure of values? *Journal of Social Issues, 50*(4), 19–45.

Smith, F. (1992). *To think: In language, learning and education.* Routledge.

Teschendorf, B., & Nemshick, M. (2001). Faculty roles in professional socialization. *Journal of Physical Therapy Education, 15,* 4–10.

Thorpe, K., & Loo, R. (2003). The values profile of nursing undergraduate students: Implications for education and professional development. *Journal of Nursing Education, 42*(2), 83–90. https://pubmed.ncbi.nlm.nih.gov/12622336/

Valutis, S., Rubin, D., & Bell, M. (2012). Professional socialization and social work values: Who are we teaching? *Social Work Education: The International Journal, 31*(8), 1046–1057. https://doi.org/10.1080/02615479.2011.610785

Wackerhausen, S. (2009). Collaboration, professional identity and reflection across boundaries. *Journal of Interprofessional Care, 23*(5), 455–473.

Weidman, J., Twale, D., & Stein, E. (2001). *Socialization of graduate and professional students in higher education: A perilous passage?* John Wiley & Sons.

Weiss, I., Gal, J., & Cnaan, R. (2004). Social work education as professional socialization: A study of the impact of social work education upon students' professional preferences. *Journal of Social Service Research, 31*(1), 13–31.

Williams, B., Spiers, J., Fisk, A., Richards, L., Gibson, B., Kabotoff, W., . . .McIlwraith, D. (2012). The influence of an undergraduate problem/context based learning program on evolving professional nursing graduate practice. *Nurse Education Today, 32*(4), 417–421. https://doi.org/10.1016/j.nedt.2011.03.002

Zarshenas, L., Sharif, F., Molazem, Z., Khayyer, M., Zare, N., & Ebadi, A. (2014). Professional socialization in nursing: A qualitative content analysis. *Iranian Journal of Nursing & Midwifery Research, 19*(4), 432–438.

6

Technology-Enhanced
Clinical Education

*Technology gives us power, but it does not and cannot tell us how to
use that power. Thanks to technology, we can instantly communicate
across the world, but it still doesn't help us know what to say.*

JONATHAN SACKS (2014, PARA 48)

Advances in technology over the past few decades have had profound
impacts on all aspects of life in North America. The practice of health
care and the education of all health-care professionals are not exceptions.
Technology for communication through email made it possible to share
information related to patient care or health professions education much
more quickly than snail mail or pneumatic tube systems. Although email
was complicated in the beginning, it became more functional with the
availability of browsers such as Internet Explorer, Firefox, and Chrome.

Once we had browsers and file sharing, electronic communication of
lab results and pharmacy prescriptions became standard within hospitals.
Still, many years passed before a hospital system could communicate with
systems outside the facility. Many hours and dollars were spent trying to
get one system to speak to another. Now, with the internet ubiquitous,
information and records can be paper free and stored in cyberspace. The
most recent advance, the smartphone, allows practitioners, students, and

educators to hold in their hands a constant connection, password-protected of course, to work or school information.

This communication technology now extends to communities, clinics, and private homes. We can now share physiological data. Patients can send their blood pressure, heart rate, cardiac rhythm, and so on via the internet to a health-care provider through what are now called wearables. Beyond needing to learn how to use these information technologies in patient care, health-care students need to learn how to use a myriad of computer-regulated equipment such as IV infusion pumps, digital scales, and cardiac monitors. The practice of health care and the basic education of practitioners must encompass understanding of and skill with technology.

In this chapter, we suggest that entry-level practice requires the use of technology. We give an overview of some common technologies and comment on how teachers need support to use technology. Describing specific strategies for clinical instruction related to all technologies is not possible here. Our intention is to uncover the possibilities for technology use in the clinical setting and to direct clinical instructors toward appropriate resources.

ENTRY-LEVEL PRACTICE REQUIRES THE USE OF TECHNOLOGY

Health-care professionals must be able to understand and use technology in the workplace. They must use information technology to assess and manage patient or client information, and they must understand the associated ethical and legal considerations. In most health professions, entry-level competencies spell out the expectations of beginning practitioners. For example, community health pharmacists have specific competency requirements for using the Electronic Health Record and the Computerized Pharmacy Management System (Accreditation Council for Canadian Physiotherapy . . . , 2009; NACDS and NCPA Task Force, 2012).

In nursing, individuals are required to be literate and competent in informatics and other communications technology. Prior to entering their program, nursing students are expected to be able to use "personal computers, tablets and mobile devices as well as other peripheral devices including USB drives and printers, . . . email, multimedia such as videos and podcasts, word processing applications, and be able to navigate operating systems such as Microsoft Windows, social media and use technology that supports self-directed learning" (Borycki & Foster, 2014, p. 15).

As an illustration of the importance of informatics, a committee of experts at the Canadian Association of Schools of Nursing (CASN) has prepared a document on nursing informatics needed for entry into practice "to promote a national dialogue among nurse educators, informatics experts, and nursing students on integrating nursing informatics into entry-to-practice competencies; to increase the capacity of Canadian nurse educators to teach nursing informatics; and to engage nursing's key stakeholders in developing nursing informatics outcome-based objectives for undergraduate nursing curricula" (CASN & CHI, 2012, p. iv).

The report titled *Nursing Informatics Indicators for Delivery of Patient Care* (CASN & CHI, 2012) identifies and demonstrates the appropriate use of a variety of information and communication technologies (ICTs)—such as point-of-care systems, electronic health records (EHR), electronic medical records (EMR), capillary blood glucose monitoring, hemodynamic monitoring, tele-homecare, and fetal heart monitoring devices—that are used to deliver safe nursing care to diverse populations in a variety of settings. A key point made in the report is that practitioners must use decision support tools (e.g., clinical alerts and reminders, critical pathways, web-based clinical practice guidelines) to assist clinical judgment and to help them provide safe patient care. It is also essential that ICTs are used in a way that supports (rather than interferes with) the client-patient relationship. The CASN and CHI report describes the various components of health information systems (e.g., results reporting, computerized provider order entry, clinical documentation, electronic medication administration records) and discusses the various types of electronic records used across the continuum of care—such as EHR, EMR, and patient health records (PHR)—and their clinical and administrative uses. The report concludes that informatics has an important role to play in improving health systems and the quality of interprofessional patient care.

More recently, in 2017, the Canadian Nurses Association and the Canadian Nursing Informatics Association formally endorsed the position statement of the International Medical Informatics Association on nursing informatics, stressing the importance of the appropriate use of ICTs in health care.

Clearly, clinical education is an appropriate arena in which to learn to use assessment tools that are moving progressively into the digital realm and to practise using digital approaches to providing care, monitoring outcomes, recording care provided, and communicating patient-related information among interdisciplinary team members. Although ethical and legal issues related to health informatics might be covered in theoretical courses, actual practice with the technologies in clinical settings can engage learners and advance their skills and knowledge related to the effective and appropriate uses of health informatics.

A Strategy to Try ▶ *How Do We Access Data?*

Although as an educator you might be very familiar with accessing the data that you need in the clinical practice area in which you teach, think about what the process looks like through the eyes of a student new to the profession or to your practice location. Make a list of the digital communication and information-gathering tools in use at the practicum site. Compare the tools on this list with those incorporated into your program's lab activities for students. If students have not been introduced to some tools, then find ways to provide additional practice time with these technologies during pre- or post-practicum conferences or during a clinical lab.

Your students will work in many different practice facilities, and most will use different technologies to access, record, and communicate patient-related data. Make sure that you are very comfortable in advance with the procedures and technologies used in each clinical practice area. Know how students will access the patient data that they require. Will students need passwords? If so, then how and when will these passwords be provided to them? Are there time (or other) limitations on when and how students can access electronic patient data? Knowing the answers to these questions and being comfortable with the procedures in advance of leading a clinical practicum will help to ease students' anxieties and allow students to proceed with confidence in relation to patient data–related technologies.

In preparation for a clinical placement in a specific facility, obtain examples of how lab work is shared electronically, samples of medication record documents, and templates for EMR. Make sure that students have the opportunity to explore these samples during simulation exercises prior to working with these tools and technologies in the clinical facility. Optimally, your faculty could establish a website that includes examples of health-related tools, templates, and technologies used in multiple health facilities, helping students to gain alternative experiences. Having actual examples and samples might not be practical for you, but you can make a mock set-up with screen shots from various clinical placements for learners to explore and practice with.

COMMON TECHNOLOGIES

Simulation

Simulation is one of the most common and widely used technologies in practicum components of postsecondary education programs. In aviation, flight deck simulators that focus on developing cognitive and psycho-motor skills have long been known to enhance pilot competence and reduce human error (Helmreich et al., 1999; Taylor et al., 2014). In business administration, simulated experiences are used to strengthen skills needed in crisis-based activities (Aertsen et al., 2013) and to support students' abilities to manage their information technology portfolios (Larson, 2013). In bioengineering, simulations help students to address challenges in understanding complex bioprocesses and systems (Roman et al., 2013).

In health care, simulation offers a safe environment for students to practise their skills and begin to adopt professional values (Shepherd et al., 2010). Since simulation can emulate the practice environment, the option of replacing required clinical hours with simulated activities has been debated for a number of years and remains contentious. Debate continues regarding whether simulated activities can or should replace contact with patients and, if so, to what extent.

Regulatory bodies usually determine the number of hours that professional programs must allocate to clinical practice. The seminal work of Hayden et al. (2014) with 10 pre-licensure programs across the United States replaced up to 50% of traditional clinical hours with simulated activities. They then assessed student competence at program end through clinical preceptor and instructor reports and pass rates on the required National Council Licensure Examination. The students were also evaluated by managers after their first six months of practice. There were no statistical differences in the preceptor, instructor, or manager ratings of students who completed traditional clinical hours and those who participated in simulated activities. The authors concluded that "substituting high-quality simulation experiences for up to half of traditional clinical hours produces comparable end-of program outcomes and new graduates that are ready for practice" (Hayden et al., 2014, p. S3).

Simulation is defined as imitation or enactment of something anticipated or in testing and as a representation of the behaviour or characteristics of one system through the use of another system, especially a computer program designed for the purpose (Dictionary.com, 2002). Using this broad definition, every activity in a clinical lab and pre- and post-practice activity could be considered a form of simulation. Systems that imitate or pretend to act as patients include actors, manikins, and different types of machines posing as patients.

In health-care education, the word *simulation* became more prominent in recent years with the development of low-, medium-, and high-fidelity manikins, artificial human patients, and artificial parts of patients that respond electronically to interventions by the learner. Clinical labs designed to teach skills to health professions use manikins programmed with realistic scenarios during practice sessions that are as close to reality as possible without a human patient being involved.

Simulation also includes low-fidelity activities such as case study discussions, role-playing interactions with patients (or other learners posing as patients), and practising skills such as changing dressings or giving injections using creative alternatives to expensive responsive computerized manikins (e.g., injecting saline into an orange or changing the dressing on a teddy bear). Many of these low-fidelity activities can be practised without actors or costly manikins to simulate patients and their conditions.

Although the introduction of high-fidelity activities has increased the opportunities for learners to practise skills in realistic emergency and specialty situations (Sharp et al., 2014), the effective use of simulation in clinical learning involves more than simply having learners use machines to practise required skills. Qualified instructors need to create and program the scenarios so that manikins exhibit realistic signs and symptoms and respond appropriately to students' interventions. These educators must effectively guide learners before, during, and after simulation experiences to maximize their learning. For example, debriefing with learners after simulation is an important part of the learning experience so that students can solidify learning, discuss their feelings and emotions, and consider alternatives to actions taken and "errors" made during simulation. Journals such as *Clinical Simulation in Nursing*, organizations such as the International Nursing Association for Clinical Simulation and Learning, and groups such as the CASN Simulation Interest Group offer valuable guidance for successfully employing a full range of simulated activities in clinical teaching.

Simulation has the potential to improve education outcomes. In health, a meta-analysis of studies related to health professions education concludes that, "in comparison with no intervention, technology-enhanced simulation training in health professions education is consistently associated with large effects for outcomes of knowledge, skills, and behaviors and moderate effects for patient-related outcomes" (Cook et al., 2011, p. 978).

Studies in medicine, paramedic training, and nursing support this conclusion. In medical education, simulators help novice surgeons to develop skills, retain knowledge, and reduce procedure times and error levels for laparoscopic surgery (Al-Kadi & Donnon, 2013). In first responder education, creating simulated accident scenes helps firefighter and paramedic students to prepare for situations that they will encounter in practice (Smith & Anderson, 2014). In nursing, simulated experiences can enhance knowledge gains (Gates et al., 2012; Shinnick et al., 2012; Weaver, 2011), decrease medication errors (Shearer, 2013), be equivalent to traditional clinical experiences promoting students' acquisition of fundamental knowledge (Hayden et al. 2014; Schlairet & Pollock, 2010), increase self-confidence (Leavett-Jones et al., 2011), and enhance efficacy (Dunn et al., 2014). However, questions remain about how these outcomes transfer to the clinical setting (Norman, 2012), whether they promote an unrealistic level of self-confidence (Liaw et al., 2012), and whether they heighten stress (Weaver 2011).

Although the nursing education literature reports many positive outcomes related to the use of simulation as part of clinical education, guidance is needed so that simulation can be used effectively and appropriately system wide. In 2015, the Canadian Association of Schools of Nursing released *Practice Domain for Baccalaureate Nursing Education: Guidelines for Clinical Placement and Simulation*. The objectives of the task force that developed the document were to identify outcome expectations, examine clinical practice and simulation in relation to these outcome expectations, and formulate principles of practice and guidelines.

There are stages of simulation. No matter what type of simulated activity educators implement, like any learning experience, simulations require detailed planning. Some learning institutions house high-fidelity simulation labs that are complex environments under the skilled leadership of dedicated simulation experts. In other instances, clinical teachers will lead students through a series of simulated activities (low or high fidelity) geared to developing specific skills. If you are a clinical educator expected to lead learners through simulated activities without the guidance of a team of experts, then we suggest seven stages that can be adapted and modified to guide most simulated activities: (1) choose or write a scenario; (2) obtain and set up equipment; (3) determine the student patterns or roles; (4) offer pre-briefing activities; (5) implement the simulation; (6) facilitate a debriefing discussion; and (7) evaluate the activity. Each stage is explained in detail below.

1. Choose or Write a Scenario

All planned learning experiences should address specific learning objectives or learning outcomes. This is no less important in a simulation. What does the instructor want the student to accomplish in the planned setting? Every simulation should have a goal, a context, and a story. These three elements should be considered whether the simulation planned is a case study in a textbook, an actor posing as a patient, a situation in the online virtual world called Second Life, or a high-fidelity simulation that uses sophisticated avatars in realistic patient care scenarios. The learning objective should thread through the simulation, allowing students to understand the goal of the simulation from the outset.

There is some debate about this point. Some educators do not want students to know the specific goal of the simulation in advance, believing that knowing the objective would reduce the impact of learning from the unknown and unexpected elements of the scenario. If as an educator you choose not to reveal the learning objective of a specific scenario to the students, then this choice (and the broad reasons for it) should be stated explicitly at the outset (Alinier, 2011; Brackney & Priode, 2015).

Once you determine your goal, you can take several routes to design your simulation. Vignettes, story boards, flowcharts, and scripts are parts of simulation pre-planning and design. These plans need to include when and where the students will receive content and context information related to the scenario. Items such as vignettes and scripts can be made by instructors, purchased from companies such as Pearson, or searched for on the internet. Many scenarios can be used freely, such as a collection of simulated situations by Reid and Raleigh (2013). As students advance in their programs, they can be invited to suggest or write their own scenarios.

2. Obtain and Set Up Equipment

Whatever the degree of fidelity, simulated activities require equipment. It could be oranges and syringes to simulate giving intramuscular injections or a complex piece of machinery such as a pediatric IV arm, with which learners can practise challenging IV initiations on a pediatric-sized artificial arm, or the NOELLE maternal care simulator, which provides learners with a complete birthing simulation experience before, during, and after delivery.

Determine the equipment that you need, practise working with it yourself, and plan the specific amount of time that each student is likely to need to complete the simulated exercise. Do you have enough time allotted (considering the group size) to ensure that everyone has sufficient time to participate fully in the exercise? If you are using low-resolution equipment (e.g., non-programmable manikins) as part of your simulation equipment, then try to humanize them as much as possible. For example, applying makeup or using other props can help to make the simulation as realistic as possible (Merica, 2011). Simply adding items such as clothing and wigs to manikins can make them seem more lifelike and consequently make the learning experience more realistic.

Bear in mind that simulated experiences do not need high fidelity. Setting up practice time with equipment that students will be using in their hospital, clinic, or community placements is also an important simulation. For example, how can you create opportunities for students to work with electronic data collection or IV pumps? One tip: it might be possible to obtain outdated equipment or supplies from health-care institutions for students to manipulate and use in practice scenarios as a form of low-cost (but realistic) simulation.

3. Determine the Student Patterns or Roles

Clinical practicum placements are now at a premium. Not every student can experience every situation or skill practice under the guidance of an instructor. This is also true in high-fidelity simulation labs. To maximize the learning, consider dividing students into groups and giving each person in the group a different role. For example, one student might actively provide care, a second might act as a consultant to the care provider, and a third could keep records. Rotate students through each role in a timely manner and ensure that all students participate in providing care during the simulation.

Johnson (2019) studied the knowledge demonstration, retention, and application of both participant and observer nurse learners during simulated experiences and concluded that there was no difference between the two roles. He advised educators to value and appreciate both roles. Instructors need to convey to learners (through their attitudes and words) the learning value of roles other than care provider. Ensure that all members of the group, no matter the role, know that there is important learning potential in participating fully.

4. Offer Pre-Briefing Activities

Pre-briefing is recognized as important in developing learners' clinical judgment and thinking. Established goals of pre-briefing activities are to support students' capacity to "notice aspects of the clinical situation, anticipate patient needs, and focus on the application of existing knowledge" (Page-Cutrara, 2014, p. 140). Students need to know why the simulation is salient and relevant to their future practice. During pre-briefing, clearly outline the learning objectives, the expectations of each role, and the times allotted to each activity. Provide any available advance reading or pre-testing activities. Review any medications that will be used during the simulation (Brackney & Priode, 2015). Specify how the simulated activity is different from real-life experience (Willett, 2013). Whenever possible, invite students to walk around the equipment and become accustomed to the space before the simulated activity begins.

5. Implement the Simulation

The Jeffries Simulation Model (Jeffries, 2005) for implementing simulated activities emphasizes having teachers offer frequent cues or directions to learners and provide ongoing feedback throughout the simulation. Expect that learners will feel anxious and self-conscious as they perform new psychomotor tasks in front of peers and others. A high-fidelity simulation can trigger discomfort (or even panic) in a student. Prior to the simulation, anticipate this possibility, and make and share a plan for students who experience uneasiness during the simulation. One approach is to establish a "safe" word that students can use to end the simulation if they experience distress.

As in the clinical situations that they are designed to illustrate, simulated activities might not progress as planned. Use opportunities when simulations go other than planned to model professionalism and critical thinking. Despite moments of stress and anxiety during the simulation, it provides learners with enhanced confidence and empowers them to be successful in real-world clinical situations if the experience is implemented by skilful educators (Baptista et al., 2016).

6. Facilitate a Debriefing Discussion

Debriefing is considered a critical component of any simulated activity (Boellaard et al., 2014; Cockerham, 2015; Fanning & Gaba, 2007; Jaye et al., 2015; Jeffries 2005; Shinnick et al., 2011; Wang et al., 2011). Ensure that time and space are available for all those who have participated in a simulated activity to share their feelings and perceptions about what occurred. In some instances, planning more time for the debriefing than for the actual simulated activity is needed.

Begin the discussion, either with students individually or in groups, by inviting them to reflect on their experience and describe (in their own words) what happened. Each student should be given the chance to speak without interruption. Follow this opening reflection by asking learners what they might do differently the next time. Emphasize how the process of balancing negative and positive reflections can strengthen clinical reasoning skills. Conclude the discussions by eliciting comments from students about how they can transfer what they learned to future real-life situations.

With larger groups, create dyads for students to share their reflections on the simulated experience with a partner. Monitor the discussions so that each partner has an equal opportunity to speak. Private reflections in the form of journal entries can also be used as a debriefing strategy. Debriefing for simulation or clinical practice is now being done online. We cover this topic more fully later in the chapter in the section on online post-conferences after real-life clinical practice.

7. Evaluate the Activity

Evaluating student performance during any simulated activity should mirror clearly established learning objectives (see Chapter 6 for an in-depth discussion of student evaluation). Psychological safety or feeling comfortable about truthfully expressing their reflections on their performance is especially important to learners during and after simulated activities (Morse, 2015; Runnacles et al., 2014). Frame evaluations within a reminder that the purpose of simulated activities is to provide opportunities for practising skills in a safe environment in which patients will not be harmed. Students need to be clear that errors are expected during simulations and that they are all opportunities for learning and for changing behaviour.

Evaluation must also include measurement of the value and usefulness of the simulated activity. Be sure to provide students with opportunities to share any recommendations for improving the simulation. A short, anonymous, online evaluation form with specific multiple-choice questions about the experience can also serve as a debriefing activity. Ensure that as the simulated experience leader you consider the students' recommendations for improvement and act on them as appropriate or possible.

A Strategy to Try ▶ *What's the Hardest Part?*

Despite the complexities in any simulated activity, when we deconstruct the process, we will likely find one or two key elements that stand out as particularly difficult and anxiety provoking. These most difficult or hardest parts might be common to most learners, or they might be individual. For example, nursing students might state that putting the needle in was the hardest part of their first intramuscular injection. Others might comment that mapping the injection site was the hardest part. Exploring what students believe is the hardest part will provide important understanding of how students approach a learning activity such as simulation. Ask them "What's the hardest part of . . . ?" When we view difficulties through the eyes of our students, we can help them to build relevant strategies to overcome specific difficulties.

Affirm that knowing what we don't know and knowing when we're wrong are positive. If something doesn't go well, then create a climate in which it's okay to be wrong. When students implement procedures and they don't go well, be sure that they know they will be supported rather than penalized for sharing what they did poorly. The important thing for students to think about is "How can I make it better?" Communicate to students that the only way they can improve and do better the next time is to discuss what they think went wrong. Genuinely let students know that you will offer feedback and guidance and that you want to hear about the times when things went wrong. Then go back into the trenches together and try again.

ADRIENNE WEARE, MN, ACADEMIC COORDINATOR, CENTRE FOR NURSING AND HEALTH STUDIES, ATHABASCA UNIVERSITY

In sum, despite the variation in fidelity among simulated activities, their purpose is to provide opportunities for learners to feel safe practising and developing their skills. Next, we discuss a sampling of additional technologies that clinical educators can use: virtual clinical labs, mobile technology, augmented reality, online post-conferencing, and social media.

VIRTUAL CLINICAL LABS

Virtual clinical labs, which also run from low to high fidelity, need to be included in any description of simulation. Licences to use these programs are generally purchased by health-care educational institutions, and individual teachers cannot use the programs in courses without those licences. Some online communities of health-care practice are really story boards with pictures and discussion questions, such as The Neighbourhood. In a licensed product called Second Life, you can find virtual clinical settings.

Technology can augment clinical experiences for students by allowing an entire group of them to feel that they are at the bedside in real time. Roving robots such as Vgo can be operated from outside the patient's room. They can record the interactions of health professionals, students, or instructors with patients as through a one-way mirror, but the technology can move with the caregiver from room to room. Vgo is not the same as video recording or using Skype because the robot is manoeuvrable from a distance, and the educator can focus on what is needed in the moment.

With Vgo, situations can also be recorded for further review by the instructor for the purpose of evaluation, by individual learners for self-reflection and learning, or by the entire class as a trigger for discussion. A patient's permission is clearly required for this type of activity, but acquiring permission does not need to be a roadblock. The Vgo is in use in hospital health education and can be used for community practice education.

A Strategy to Try ▶ *Visit a Virtual Clinical Lab*
Find out whether the program in which you teach has access to any virtual clinical lab. If access is available, then visit the lab and identify two or three cases or scenarios that are relevant to your clinical area. Create links between virtual cases and real-life cases in the clinical practice area.

MOBILE TECHNOLOGY

Mobile technology that incorporates information, decision platforms, and communication ability for expert advice is becoming ubiquitous in most health-care practice. Unfortunately, cellphones are stigmatized in some areas of health profession education and practice. Concerns relate to disease transmission (if the device becomes contaminated, then it can transfer bacteria or viruses from patient to patient), privacy, and possibility of inappropriate use. These concerns can all be mitigated with appropriate care and use of these devices.

The reality is that mobile technology use is ubiquitous (including in health-care settings), and the benefits (e.g., being able to check drug dosages from a patient's bedside) are compelling. Health-care professional education needs to incorporate knowledge about the ethical and appropriate use of mobile technology in health-care settings. Topics should include how to maintain appropriate infection control strategies and issues related to patients' privacy and confidentiality when using mobile technology as part of their care.

Health-care professionals commonly use hand-held devices, particularly smartphones, to replace textbooks and traditional references such as pocket formularies. Commercial software with mix-and-match selections of products is becoming popular. A Canadian study assessing the self-efficacy of nursing faculty and student use of mobile technology indicated that both faculty members and students are highly confident in their use of mobile technology and prepared to engage in mobile learning (Kenny et al., 2012). Professionals value having the information that they need at the point of care as they make critical decisions about patient care (Lamarche & Park, 2012).

The possibilities for clinical teachers to connect with their students through smartphone apps are limitless. Students can access links to relevant resources, homework assignments, or even examinations on their phones. Some instructors use smartphone connections to communicate with students during their clinical placements. For example, with a ratio of 1 instructor to 8 learners, an instructor cannot physically be with all learners at one time. Students can message their instructor when they need supervision with a skill or if they need other support or assistance in the learning experience and to help enhance patients' safety.

Other instructors use smartphone connections with learners to transmit timely motivational messages related to their learning journeys or to convey important details about upcoming learning opportunities. In an Australian study, clinical nurse educators uploaded presentations, videos, quizzes, case studies, and discussion boards weekly to promote action-oriented learning (O'Neill et al., 2018). They found that this mobile strategy increased nurses' knowledge, promoted active engagement of learners, encouraged technology use, and improved clinical practice.

Mobile technology is currently part of the teaching and learning of students in the health professions and an increasingly common (and useful) tool at the point of care for practising professionals. It is essential that educators learn to use mobile technology effectively and appropriately and include it in the curricula for health professionals.

Instructors can use texting to communicate with their students. One concern about texting is that messages might not be considered urgent. Students might think that texts can just be ignored until an appropriate time to view them. Another concern is about privacy. Both instructors and students must consent to share their phone numbers for this purpose. At the beginning of a clinical practicum, establish the ground rules for using (or not using) texting throughout the rotation.

AUGMENTED REALITY

Augmented reality (AR) is a new set of technologies that provides "a means of delivering additional content on-demand, at the point of encounter with an object in the physical world" (Garrett et al., 2018). Common examples of AR in society include technology that allows consumers to try on clothes virtually, see how they look in a new hairstyle, or view how furniture looks in their homes.

Using image recognition or location recognition technologies, physical objects or places in the world are identified and then augmented with digital information. People can view the augmented objects through head-mounted eyewear, a glass transparent screen, or a camera display such as on a smartphone or tablet (Garrett et al., 2018). It is important to note that AR does not provide opportunities for interacting with the objects (at least not at this point).

Via a smartphone, tablet, or other mobile device, AR provides students and practitioners in the health professions with multimedia networked references (including sound, video, and geographical data) that they can use to understand what medical procedures or pieces of equipment look like and how to implement them safely and appropriately.

Canadian research exploring the use of AR with nursing students (Garrett et al., 2015), and with physical therapy and occupational therapy students (Garrett et al., 2018), determined that introducing AR resources in clinical skills lab experiences helped students to create conceptual links to the physical equipment that they would use in practice. These researchers chose or created 126 different AR resources that included instructional materials with multimedia content. The resources were easy to use, and they provided opportunities for problem solving. Examples included how to perform clinical hand washing and how to operate a ceiling lift safely (Garrett et al., 2018).

The selected resources were hosted on a university web server and then linked to mobile devices through a Junaio application with associated Metaio backend service (Garrett et al., 2018). Students and instructors scanned the resources to their smartphones or devices. Therefore, they were able to review the selected multimedia content during their clinical lab experiences or at any time on their own. Students gained immediate access to digital multimedia that showed them how the equipment that they would use in clinical practice worked, explained its theoretical context, and provided instruction on how to use the equipment (Garrett et al., 2018).

Additional AR resources that Bernie Garrett and his team of researchers implemented included material specific to students' clinical placements. Prior to attending their clinical sites, students could scan in an AR resource that included a description of their clinical unit, contact information for key staff members (email and telephone), clothes-changing and parking facilities available, and transportation options to the site (Garrett et al., 2018).

AR resources cannot be expected to replace the personal instruction that occurs particularly during instructor-led demonstrations. However, it is important for clinical teachers to locate AR resources that are relevant and to integrate them into their instruction. Many students value mobile devices and appreciate using them to support their active and self-directed learning.

A Strategy to Try ▶ *Look What I Found! An AR Resource Show and Tell*
Invite students to find and curate new AR resources that would be helpful in their learning or clinical practice. Host a "show and tell" session during which students demonstrate the resources that they have acquired to their classmates and describe the uses, limitations, and benefits of each. Have the group choose a "winner" or "winners" in categories such as the most innovative innovation, the most useful resource, the most simple to explain, the most beneficial, et cetera.

ONLINE POST-CONFERENCING

Whether after an orchestrated clinical simulation or an 8-hour clinical experience in a clinic or hospital, there is great value in a debriefing session. Traditionally, these debriefing sessions have been held immediately after the experience, in a face-to-face environment close to where the learning experience occurred. The students (usually 8–10) are required to reflect on and ask questions about the experience of the day and share what they learned and what they felt.

Recently, technology such as asynchronous learning management systems has made it possible to postpone clinical post-conferencing until a time when the learner is rested and has had a chance to think about what happened during the learning experience. Online post-conferencing has many pedagogical advantages, such as demonstrating deeper learning (Bristol & Kyarsgaard, 2012). Learners can also participate at their own pace when they feel ready, so it is more convenient and flexible. Additionally, those who are shy to speak up in face-to-face environments often feel more comfortable participating in an online milieu.

As learners post their reflections online, and then respond to their colleagues and interact with one another, a collaborative learning environment with peer support and a sense of community is created (Berkstresser, 2016). Learners are not only gaining valuable knowledge about theory and practice but also developing team skills and learning about professional relationship development (Ebersole-Berkstresser, 2013). Self-motivated learners participate fully in an asynchronous online discussion moderated by the clinical or simulation instructor and gain knowledge and confidence that can be helpful in the clinical practice environment.

A Strategy to Try ▶ *Compare and Share*

Ask students who are currently in clinical practice settings to participate in an online post-conference after one practice experience and to participate in a face-to-face post-conference after a second clinical experience. Next invite students to write a short reflection comparing their experiences with the two post-conference formats.

Summarize the themes that emerge from the students' reflections. Are there any lessons learned that you can use as an educator to maximize the learning value of the clinical post-conference for this group of learners?

SOCIAL MEDIA

Social media refer to interactive internet platforms in which users create, share, and exchange information in online communities. Facebook, Twitter, Instagram, and LinkedIn are well-known social media programs. Students use social media widely in their free time, particularly those who are younger (Tuominen et al., 2014). Social media platforms hold promise as important teaching tools in clinical education. Students have gained important insights from creating a professional presence on social media, blogging on clinical topics, contributing to Wikipedia, using wikis for collaborative group work, and sharing their presentations on SlideShare, Slide Rocket, Glogster, or Prezi (Schmitt et al., 2012). Some educators might have limited experience with social media platforms, but the use of these platforms in higher education has been steadily increasing (Seaman & Tinti-Kane, 2013).

Note that, though students might use social media platforms extensively, they might not understand professional nuances of privacy and ethics on those platforms (Grajales et al., 2014; Schmitt et al., 2012; Thompson et al., 2011). Problems identified among health-care learners include separating personal and professional identities (DeCamp et al., 2013), posting photographs of interactions with identifiable patients (Thompson et al., 2011), and using informal or colloquial language in their public communications (Killam et al., 2013).

The Canadian Nurses Association (2012) provides guidance on the use of social media in its seminal publication *When Private Becomes Public: The Ethical Challenges and Opportunities of Social Media*. This publication covers rules, social norms, and etiquette for using social media in the health-care setting, outlines ethical challenges, emphasizes that patient confidentiality and privacy must be maintained if social media are used, and acknowledges that social media can be an effective tool for nurses to become influential in issues related to social justice. Most fundamental is the reminder that social media by their nature are public, and users should not consider them private in any way.

Although there is positive potential for social media in health-care education and practice, educators, learners, and practitioners need to use them with skill and knowledge. Educators have an important role in conveying this, but first they must become competent themselves. The stakes are high, especially related to ethical and privacy issues, if slip-ups are made using social media in health care.

A Strategy to Try ▶ *Now That's Professional*

Invite students to review online profiles of faculty members or professional staff members working in the clinical area in which they hope to practise after graduating. Have students identify one or two specific aspects of the profile that they would like to emulate on their own present or future professional website.

Discuss what drew students to these aspects of the profile and why they stood out as professional. How did the author of the profile use (or not use) words and pictures intentionally and appropriately? Which precautions were put in place to ensure privacy?

A Strategy to Try ▶ *Analyze a Twitter Feed*

Have students follow a health-care leader or administrator in their field on Twitter. Ask them to conduct an analysis of the person's Twitter feed, comparing the posts to the rules, social norms, and etiquette discussed in the Canadian Nurses Association (2012) publication. Did the person use social media to influence issues such as social justice?

TEACHERS NEED SUPPORT TO USE TECHNOLOGY

Using technology can be challenging. Clinical teachers need support as they sort through all of the options and possibilities available. Several tensions come with using new technologies in teaching. How do clinical educators, with years of practice and experience, find creative ways to capitalize on the new digital and networked technologies and simulated activities, particularly if they were not exposed to them in their own education? How do educators remain relevant when students can learn independently (with the right technology) because the classroom can be "anywhere, anytime, anyhow"?

Other tensions for educators come from shifts in educational philosophies (see Chapter 2). Many institutions of higher education now espouse shifting away from a traditional liberal philosophy emphasizing methods of transmission or demonstration. Instead, many health-care education programs are now embracing a more constructivist approach in which teachers build upon what students already know (Melrose et al., 2013). In such a shift, learners take increasing responsibility for their learning (often using technology as their "teachers"), and educators have to rethink their roles.

Connectivist approaches are becoming popular. Students recognize what they need to know, use the abundance of digital networks and resources to gather information, and then organize this content in useful ways (Melrose et al., 2013). Perhaps the new role for educators is less that of the gatekeeper and dispenser of information and more that of the person who guides learners in the morals, ethics, and etiquette of technology use for professional practitioners. For example, questions about the credibility of sources used by students might not have straightforward answers (Keir et al., 2018), and helping learners to find these answers can be one skill that educators can focus on during this time of role transition.

Students and practitioners have long been expected to participate in collaborative projects and develop communities of practice (Lave & Wenger, 1991; Wenger, 1998; Wenger et al., 2002). Access to these communities is no longer restricted by time and place. Students can connect digitally with like-minded others from around the world at any time and in a variety of new ways. Group work has also changed dramatically with the implementation of technological communication tools that allow learners to communicate synchronously or asynchronously on the same document or presentation.

With the increased possibilities for virtual working and connecting comes the need for new skills of collaboration that can also be guided by skilled educators. When clinical teachers engage with students online, it is often by example that they teach students how to collaborate and build a community online. When an instructor establishes a positive online learning environment, nurtures an inclusive community, and develops a supportive rapport with learners, that instructor role-models these skills of collaboration and team building (Farmer & Ramsdale, 2016).

In Chapter 3, we discussed intergenerational learners, noting how individuals in their 20s and 30s (Millennials) and those born after 1995 (Generation Zers) have grown up with technology. Those in their 40s (Generation Xers) and in their middle years (Baby Boomers) might (or might not) be less comfortable with technology. For those less familiar and comfortable with digital innovations, the technology can be confusing and even annoying. If the pedagogical purpose of a program, app, or simulation is not clear, then educators must raise questions about its use. Neither students nor teachers have time to spare on technologies just for the novelty of using them.

On a practical level, administrative support for teachers to implement new technologies can be limited. Funding and release time for them to attend workshops and learn how to use equipment themselves might not be available (Goldsworthy, 2012; Jeffries, 2008). Most technologies, particularly those offering high-fidelity simulation experiences, are expensive and might be shared among different learning programs. Schedules might provide only minimal time for learners to access equipment (Garrett et al., 2011). Space for critically important post-simulation discussion and debriefing might not be provided.

Jeffries (2008) used the acronym STEP to propose a sequence of steps that can help to create the support that instructors need to implement simulation activities confidently. These steps apply to all learning technologies. S is for standardized material and suggests initiating and maintaining a repository of easily accessible materials about simulation for all educators. T is for training the trainers and encourages health-care faculties to promote education for instructors, for example designating a champion or individual with expertise to promote the simulated activities. E is for understanding the importance of top-down encouragement. Teams can be developed to work on a plan for introducing simulation education for instructors. An orientation plan and guidelines need to be developed and shared. And P is for the planning itself and suggests ongoing collaborative activities such as forming an interest group for clinical teachers and any interested instructors.

A Strategy to Try ▶ *Step Up for Simulation*

Consider whether one, two, or even all of the strategies that Jeffries (2008) suggests in her STEP model might be useful to you.

S (repository of standardized material). Start a repository by collecting and then posting journal articles related to simulation on an interfaculty website.

T (train the trainer). Consider the idea of championing simulation. Would you be interested in taking on this role? Could you co-create a champion role with another teacher interested in simulation?

E (top-down encouragement). How can you contribute to any orientation or guideline for implementing simulated activities that already are, or should be, in place? Can you extend existing processes to be more team oriented?

P (planning). If a simulation interest group is not in place in your training program, can you initiate one? Can you make links between program interest groups and national interest groups such as the CASN Simulation Interest Group?

CONCLUSION

In this chapter, we discussed how technology can enhance clinical education. To achieve entry-level competencies, students in the health professions must use technology. We provided an overview of common technologies, elaborating on simulation. We emphasized that the purpose of simulated activities is to provide safe environments in which students can practise the skills that they need to learn. Whether simulation is a low-fidelity activity such as discussing a written case study or a high-fidelity activity such as operating a complex machine simulating a human function, students need supportive feedback throughout the activity. Establishing a climate in which it is acceptable to be wrong (and to learn from the error) is an essential element of any simulated activity. Time and space must be available at the end of a simulation to debrief and reflect critically on how the activity developed.

Virtual clinical labs, mobile technology, augmented reality, online post-conferencing, and social media are additional technologies that can enhance clinical teaching. As with the use of any innovation, teachers themselves might need support in learning how to use the technology before they can be effective in guiding learners to use it ethically, appropriately, and effectively.

REFERENCES

Accreditation Council for Canadian Physiotherapy Academic Programs, Canadian Alliance of Physiotherapy Regulators, Canadian Physiotherapy Association, Canadian Council of Physiotherapy University Programs. (2009). *Essential Competency Profile for Physiotherapists in Canada*. http://www.physiotherapyeducation.ca/Resources/Essential%20Comp%20PT%20Profile%202009.pdf

Aertsen, T., Jaspaert, K., & Van Gorp, B. (2013). From theory to practice: A crisis simulation exercise. *Business Communication Quarterly, 76*(3), 322–338. https://doi.org/10.1177/1080569913482575

Alinier, A. (2011). A guide for developing high-fidelity simulation scenarios in healthcare education and continuing professional development. *Simulation & Gaming, 42*(1), 9–26. http://uhra.herts.ac.uk/bitstream/handle/2299/9334/904785.pdf?sequence=1

Al-Kadi, A. S., & Donnon, T. (2013). Using simulation to improve the cognitive and psychomotor skills of novice students in advanced laparoscopic surgery: A meta-analysis. *Medical Teacher, 35,* S47–S55. https://doi.org/10.3109/0142159X.2013.765549

Baptista, R., Pereira, F., & Martins, J. (2016). Perception of nursing students on high-fidelity practices. *Journal of Nursing Education and Practice, 6*(8), 10–21. https://pdfs.semanticscholar.org/e142/4c142c70974fa07a6533098a85ed2d56110d.pdf

Berkstresser, K. (2016). The use of online discussions for post-clinical conference. *Nurse Education in Practice, 16*(1), 27–32. https://doi.org/10.1016/j.nepr.2015.06.007

Boellaard, C., Brandt, C., Johnson, N., & Zorn, C. (2014). Practicing for practice: Accelerated second baccalaureate degree nursing (ABSN) students evaluate simulations. *Nursing Education Perspectives, 35*(4), 257–258.

Borycki, E., & Foster, J. (2014). A comparison of Australian and Canadian informatics competencies for undergraduate nurses. In K. Saranto et al. (Eds.), *Nursing informatics*, IOS Press. http://eprints.qut.edu.au/77800/1/77800.pdf

Brackney, E., & Priode, E. (2015). Creating context with prebriefing: A case example using simulation. *Journal of Nursing Education and Practice, 5*(1), 129–136.

Bristol, T. J., & Kyarsgaard, V. (2012). Asynchronous discussion: A comparison of larger and smaller discussion group size. *Nursing Education Perspectives, 33*(6), 386–390. https://doi.org/10.5480/1536-5026-33.6.386

Canadian Association of Schools of Nursing. (2015). *Practice domains for baccalaureate nursing education: Guidelines for clinical placement and simulation*. https://www.casn.ca/wp-content/uploads/2015/11/Draft-clinical-sim-2015.pdf

Canadian Association of Schools of Nursing and Canada Health Infoway. (2012). *Nursing informatics: Entry-to-practice competencies for registered nurses*. http://www.casn.ca/2014/12/nursing-informatics-entry-practice-competencies-registered-nurses-2/

Canadian Nurses Association. (2012). *When private becomes public: The ethical challenges and opportunities of social media.* Ethics in Practice for Registered Nurses. Professional Practice and Regulation division of the CNA publication. https://www.cna-aiic.ca/~/media/cna/page-content/pdf-en/ethics_in_practice_feb_2012_e.pdf?la=en

Cockerham, M. E. (2015). Effect of faculty training on improving the consistency of student assessment and debriefing in clinical simulation. *Clinical Simulation in Nursing, 11*(1), 64–71. https://doi.org/10.1016/j.ecns.2014.10.011

Cook, D., Brydges, R., Zendejas, B., Szostek, J. A., Erwin, S., & Hamstra, S. (2011). Technology-enhanced simulation for health professions education: A systematic review and meta-analysis. *The Journal of the American Medical Association, 306*(9), 978–988.

DeCamp, M., Koenig, T., & Chisolm, M. (2013). Social media and physician's online identity crisis. *The Journal of the American Medical Association, 310*(6), 581–582.

Dictionary.com. (2002). Simulation. https://www.dictionary.com/browse/simulation

Dunn, K., Osborne, C., & Link, H. (2014). High-fidelity simulation and nursing student self-efficacy: Does training help the little engines know they can? *Nursing Education Perspectives, 35*(6), 403–404. https://doi.org/10.5480/12-1041.1

Ebersole-Berkstresser, K. A. (2013). *Online clinical post-conference, face-to-face clinical post-conference: Effects on critical thinking in associate degree nursing students* (Unpublished doctoral dissertation). Capella University, Minneapolis, MN.

Fanning, R., & Gaba, D. (2007). The role of debriefing in simulation-based learning. *Simulation in Healthcare, 2*(2), 115–125.

Farmer, H. M., & Ramsdale, J. (2016). Teaching competencies for the online environment. *Canadian Journal of Learning & Technology, 42*(3), 1. https://doi.org/10.21432/T2V32J

Garrett, B., Anthony, J., & Jackson, C. (2018). Using mobile augmented reality to enhance health professional practice education. *Current Issues in Emerging E-Learning, 4*(1), Art. 10. https://scholarworks.umb.edu/ciee/vol4/iss1/10

Garrett, B. M., Jackson, C. & Wilson, B. (2015). Augmented reality m-learning to enhance nursing skills acquisition in the clinical skills laboratory. *Interactive Technology and Smart Education, 12* (4), 298–314. https://doi.org/ 10.1108/ITSE-05-2015-0013

Garrett, B., MacPhee, M., & Jackson, C. (2011). Implementing high-fidelity simulation in Canada: Reflections on 3 years of practice. *Nursing Education Today, 31*(7), 671–676. https://doi.org/10.1016/j.nedt.2010.10.028

Gates, M., Parr, M., & Hughen, J. (2012). Enhancing nursing knowledge using high-fidelity simulation. *Journal of Nursing Education, 51*(1), 9–15.

Goldsworthy, S. (2012). High fidelity simulation in critical care: A Canadian perspective. *Collegian, 19*(3), 139–143. https://doi.org/10.1016/j.colegn.2012.06.003

Grajales, F., Sheps, S., Ho, K., Novak-Lauscher, H., & Eysenbach, G. (2014). Social media: A review and tutorial of applications in medicine and health care. *Journal of Medical Internet Research, 16*(2): e13. https://doi.org/10.2196/jmir.2912

Hayden, J. K., Smiley, R. A., Alexander, M., Kardong-Edgren, S., & Jeffries, P. R. (2014). The NCSBN national simulation study: A longitudinal, randomized, controlled study replacing clinical hours with simulation in prelicensure nursing education. *Journal of Nursing Regulation, 5*(2), 1–66.

Helmreich, R. L., Merritt, A. C., & Wilhelm, J. A. (1999). The evolution of crew resource management training in commercial aviation. *International Journal of Aviation Psychology, 9*(1), 19–32.

Jaye, P., Thomas, L., & Reedy, G. (2015). "The Diamond": A structure for simulation debrief. *The Clinical Teacher, 12*, 171–175.

Jeffries, P. R. (2005). A framework for designing, implementing, and evaluating simulations used as teaching strategies in nursing. *Nursing Education Perspectives, 26*(2), 28–35.

Jeffries, p. (2008). Getting in S.T.E.P. with simulations: Simulations take educator preparation. *Nursing Education Perspectives, 29*(2), 70–73.

Johnson, B. (2019). Simulation observers learn the same as participants: The evidence. *Simulation in Nursing, 33*, 26–34.

Keir, A., Bamat, N., Patel, R., Elkhateeb, O., & Roland, D. (2018). Utilising social media to educate and inform healthcare professionals, policy makers and the broader community. *British Medical Journal, 24*(3), 87–89.

Kenny, R., Van Neste-Kenny, J., Burton, P., Park, C., & Qayyum, A. (2012). Using self-efficacy to assess the readiness of nursing educators and students for mobile learning. *The International Review of Research in Open and Distributed Learning, 13*(3), 277–296. http://www.irrodl.org/index.php/irrodl/article/view/1221

Killam, L., Carter, L., & Graham, R. (2013). Facebook and issues of professionalism in undergraduate nursing education: Risky business or risk worth taking? *International Journal of E-Learning and Distance Education, 27*(2), 1–22.

Lamarche, K., & Park, C. (2012). The views of nurse practitioner students on the value of personal digital assistants in clinical practice. *Canadian Journal of Nursing Informatics, 7*(1). http://cjni.net/journal/?p=1962

Larson, E. (2013). Teaching tip utilizing classroom simulation to convey key concepts in IT portfolio management. *Journal of Information Systems Education, 24*(2), 99–104.

Lave, J., & Wenger, E. (1991). *Situated learning: Legitimate peripheral participation.* Cambridge University Press.

Levett-Jones, T., Lapkin, S., Hoffman, K., Arthur, C., & Roche, J. (2011). Examining the impact of high and medium fidelity simulation experiences on nursing students' knowledge acquisition. *Nurse Education in Practice, 11*(6), 380–383. https://doi.org/10.1016/j.nepr.2011.03.014

Liaw, S., Scherpbier, A., Rethans, J., & Klainin-Yobas, p. (2012). Assessment for simulation learning outcomes: A comparison of knowledge and self-reported confidence with observed clinical performance. *Nurse Education Today, 32*(6), e35–e39.

Melrose, S., Park, C., & Perry, B. (2013). *Teaching health professionals online: Frameworks and strategies*. Athabasca University Press. http://www.aupress.ca/index. php/books/120234

Merica, B. (2011). *Medical moulage: How to make your simulations come alive*. F. A. Davis.

Morse, K. (2015). Structured model of debriefing on perspective transformation for NP students. *Clinical Simulation in Nursing, 11*(3), 172–179. https://doi. org/10.1016/j.ecns.2015.01.001

NACDS and NCPA Task Force. (2012). *Entry-level competencies needed for community pharmacy practice*. https://www.acpe-accredit.org/pdf/NACDSFoundation- NCPA-ACPETaskForce2012.pdf

Norman, J. (2012). Systematic review of the literature on simulation in nursing education. *Association of Black Nursing Faculty, 23*(2), 24–26.

O'Neill, K., Robb, M., Kennedy, R., Bhattacharya, A., Dominici, N. R., & Murphy, A. (2018). Mobile technology, just-in-time learning and gamification: Innovative strategies for a CAUTI education program. *Online Journal of Nursing Informatics, 22*(2). https://www.himss.org/resources/mobile-technology-just-time-learning- and-gamification-innovative-strategies-cauti

Page-Cutrara, K. (2014). Use of prebriefing in nursing simulation: A literature review. *Journal of Nursing Education, 53*(3), 136–141. https://doi.org/10.3928/ 01484834-20140211-07

Reid, C., & Raleigh, R. (2013). *Where to find simulation scenarios*. Riverland Community College. http://www.riverland.edu/mnsim/Where%20to%20find% 20Simulation%20Scenarios.pdf

Roman, M., Popescu, D., & Selişteanu, D. (2013). An interactive teaching system for bond graph modeling and simulation in bioengineering. *Educational Technology & Society, 16*(4), 17–31.

Runnacles, J., Thomas, L., Sevdalis, N., Kneebone, R., & Arora, S. (2014). Development of a tool to improve performance debriefing and learning: The paediatric Objective Structured Assessment of Debriefing (OSAD) tool. *Postgrad Medical Journal, 90*(1069), 613–621. https://doi.org/10.1136/postgrad medj-2012-131676

Sacks, J. (2014). *On creative minorities*. The 2013 Erasmus Lecture. https://www. firstthings.com/article/2014/01/on-creative-minorities

Schlairet, M., & Pollock, J. (2010). Equivalence testing of traditional and simulated clinical experiences: Undergraduate nursing students' knowledge acquisition. *Journal of Nursing Education, 49*(1), 43–47.

Schmitt, T., Sims-Giddens, S., & Booth, R. (2012). Social media use in nursing education. *The Online Journal of Issues in Nursing, 17*(3), Ms. 2. https://doi.org/10.3912/ OJIN.Vol17No03Man02

Seaman, J., & Tinti-Kane, H. (2013). *Social media for teaching and learning*. Pearson Learning Solutions.

Sharp, P., Newberry, L., Fleishauer, M., & Doucette, J. (2014). High-fidelity simulation and its impact in the acute care setting. *Nursing Management, 45*(7), 32–39.

Shearer, J. (2013). High fidelity simulation and safety: An integrative review. *Journal of Nursing Education, 52*(1), 39–45.

Shepherd, C., McCunnis, M., Brown, L., & Hair, M. (2010). Investigating the use of simulation as a teaching strategy. *Nursing Standard, 24*(35), 42–48.

Shinnick, M., Woo, M., & Evangelista, L. (2012). Predictors of knowledge gains using simulation in the education of prelicensure nursing students. *Journal of Professional Nursing, 28*(1), 41–47.

Shinnick, M. A., Woo, M., Horwich, T. B., & Steadman, R. (2011). Debriefing: The most important component in simulation? *Clinical Simulation in Nursing, 7*(3), e105–e111. https://doi.org/lo.1016/j.ecns.2010.11.005

Smith, A., & Andersen, p. (2014). Proven effective: Simulation-based assessment facilitates learning & enhances clinical judgment. *Journal of Emergency Medical Services, Suppl.*, 3–8.

Taylor, A., Dixon-Hardy, D., & Wright, S. (2014). Simulation training in U.K. general aviation: An undervalued aid to reducing loss of control accidents. *International Journal of Aviation Psychology, 24*(2), 141–152.

Thompson, L., Black, E., Duff, W., Paradise Black, N., Saliba, H., & Dawson, K. (2011). Protected health information on social networking sites: Ethical and legal considerations. *Journal of Medical Internet Research, 13*(1), e8. https://doi.org/10.2196/jmir.1590

Tuominen, R., Stolt, M., & Salminen, L. (2014). Social media in nursing education: The view of the students. *Education Research International*, Article ID 929245, 1–6. https://doi.org/10.1155/2014/929245

Wang, E. E., Kharasch, M., & Kuruna, D. (2011). Facilitative debriefing techniques for simulation-based learning. *Academic Emergency Medicine, 18*, e5. https://doi.org/10.1111/j.1553-2712.2010.01001.x

Weaver, A. (2011). High-fidelity patient simulation in nursing education: An integrative review. *Nursing Education Perspectives, 32*(1), 37–40. https://doi.org/10.5480/1536-5026-32.1.37

Wenger, E. (1998). *Communities of practice: Learning, meaning and identity.* Cambridge University Press.

Wenger, E., McDermott, R., & Snyder, W. (2002). *Cultivating communities of practice.* Harvard Business School Press.

Willett, T. (2013). *Pre-brief design is crucial* [Fact sheet]. Tip #351, SIM-One—The Ontario Simulation Network. http://www.sim-one.ca/community/tip/pre-brief-design-crucial

7

Evaluation of Learning

Ever tried. Ever failed. No matter.
Try Again. Fail again. Fail better.
SAMUEL BECKETT (1983, P. 11)

Few topics generate more impassioned discussions among educators of health-care professionals than the evaluation of learning. In many clinical practice settings, instructors are required to apply tools of evaluation that they have not designed themselves. On the one hand, criticisms of standardized assessment techniques for required professional competencies and skill sets note the overemphasis on reproducing facts by rote or implementing memorized procedures. On the other, teachers might find themselves filling out extensive and perhaps incomprehensible checklists of criteria intended to measure critical thinking. How can evaluation possibilities be created to advance required competencies with individuals in complex practice environments?

Expectations of learners must be set out clearly before learning can be measured accurately. Within the clinical environment, the stakes are high for learners. Client safety cannot be compromised. Furthermore, measurement considerations must not dominate the time that educators might otherwise spend on creating meaningful instructional approaches. In his seminal *Learning to Teach in Higher Education*, Paul Ramsden (1992) establishes an important distinction between *deep* learning and *surface* learning. In his view, deep and meaningful learning occurs when assessment focuses on both what students need to learn and how educators can best teach them.

Understanding the complexities of evaluating students and our teaching is an ongoing process. Approaching the process collaboratively in ways that consistently involve learners as active participants, rather than passive recipients, can support their success and inspire our teaching. In this chapter, we introduce the vocabulary of evaluation and discuss methods of evaluating both students and teachers. We suggest creative strategies for evaluation that teachers can use in a variety of clinical practice settings.

VOCABULARY OF EVALUATION

Educators can feel overwhelmed by measuring how learners create personal meaning and demonstrate understanding of the consensually validated knowledge that they will need to practise competently in their health fields. Measuring the efficacy of our own teaching in relation to preparing learners to practise safely, ethically, and in accordance with entry-to-practice competencies is not straightforward either. However, whether we are seeking to appraise student learning or our own teaching, knowing the criteria for expected outcomes will help us to understand what is being measured. The terms "measurement," "assessment," "evaluation," "feedback," and "grading" are used in appraising student learning and our own teaching.

Measurement, Assessment, and Evaluation

Measurement determines the attributes of a physical object in relation to a standard instrument. For example, just as a thermometer measures temperature, so too standardized educational tests measure student performance. Reliable and valid measurement depends on the skilful use of appropriate and accurate instruments. In 1943, Douglas Scales was one of the first to argue against applying the principles of scientific measurement to the discipline of education.

The kind of science that seeks only the simplest generalizations can depart rather far from flesh-and-blood reality, but the kind of science that can be applied in the everyday work of teachers, administrators, and counsellors must recognize the great variety of factors in the practical conditions under which these people do their work. Any notion of science that stems from a background of engineering concepts in which all significant variables can be readily identified, isolated, measured, and controlled is both inadequate and misleading. Education, in both its theory and its practice, requires a new perspective in science that will enable it to deal with composite phenomena in which physical science normally deals with highly specific, single factors (Scales, 1943, p. 1).

One example of a standardized measurement tool is a required student evaluation form. Most health profession programs provide clinical instructors with evaluation forms designed to measure learning outcomes in relation to course objectives. These forms provide standardization in that they are implemented with all students in a course. They often focus on competencies such as safety, making them relevant to all members of the profession (Walsh et al., 2010). However, clinical instructors who use the forms might have little or no input into their construction and might not see clear links to their own practice setting.

Another example of a standardized measurement tool is a qualifying examination that all members of a profession must pass in order to practise. Similarly, skills competency checklists, rating scales, multiple choice tests, and medication dosage calculation quizzes can provide standardized measurement. Again, clinical instructors might have limited input into the design of these tools.

Assessment obtains information in relation to a complex objective, goal, or outcome. Although the standardized measurements noted above can all contribute to assessing student performance, additional information is necessary. Processes for assessment require inferences about what individuals do in relation to what they know (Assessment, n.d.). For example, inferences can be drawn about how students apply theory to practice from instructors' observations of students while implementing client care, from student self-assessments, and from peer assessments.

Evaluation makes judgments about value or worth in relation an objective, goal, or outcome. Evaluation needs information from a variety of sources and at different times. Evaluation of learners in clinical practice settings is considered subjective rather than objective (Emerson, 2007; Gaberson et al., 2015; Gardner & Suplee, 2010; O'Connor, 2015).

Formative evaluation is continuous, diagnostic, and focused on both what students are doing well and what they need to improve (Carnegie Mellon, n.d.). Because the goal of formative evaluation is to improve future performance, a mark or grade is not usually included (Gaberson et al., 2015; Marsh et al., 2005). Formative evaluation, sometimes referred to as mid-term evaluation, should precede final or summative evaluation.

Summative evaluation summarizes how students have or have not achieved the outcomes and competencies stipulated in course object-ives (Carnegie Mellon, n.d.) and includes a mark or grade. Summative evaluation can be completed at mid-term or end of term. Both formative evaluation and summative evaluation consider context. They can include measurement and assessment methods noted previously as well as staff observations, written work, presentations, and a variety of other measures.

Whether the term "measurement," "assessment," or "evaluation" is used, the outcome criteria or what is expected must be defined clearly and measured fairly. The process must be transparent and consistent. For all those who teach and learn in health-care fields, succeeding or not succeeding has profound consequences.

A Strategy to Try ▶ *The Experience of Being Judged*
Clinical teachers measure (quantify), assess (infer), and evaluate (judge). Tune in to a time in your own learning or practice when your performance was measured. The experience of having others who are in positions of power over us make inferences and judgments about what we know can be both empowering and disempowering. Reflect on an occasion when you were evaluated. Did the evaluation offer a balanced view of your strengths and weaknesses? Did you find yourself focusing more on the weaknesses than on the strengths? How can our own experiences with being judged help us to be better teachers?

Students also bring with them experiences of being judged. One helpful strategy might be to have them share their best and worst experiences of evaluation. Focus a discussion on the factors that made this their best or worst experience to help learners reveal their fears. You can consider asking learners to draw a picture of their experience before they reflect on and discuss it.

Feedback

Feedback differs from assessment and evaluation. Assessment requires instructors to make inferences, and evaluation requires them to make judgments. Feedback is defined as "a process through which learners make sense of information from various sources and use it to enhance their work or learning strategies" (Carless & Boud, 2018, p. 1315). Feedback is non-judgmental and requires instructors to provide learners with information that facilitates improvement (Concordia University, n.d.). Feedback should focus on tasks rather than on individuals, it should be specific, and it should be directly linked to learners' personal goals (Archer, 2010).

Periodic, timely, constructive feedback that recognizes both strengths and areas for improvement is perceived by students as encouraging and helpful in bolstering their confidence and independence (Bradshaw & Lowenstein, 2014). The tone of verbal or written feedback should always communicate respect for the student and for any work done. The feedback should be specific enough that students know what to do but not so specific that the work is done for them (Brookhart, 2008).

Chickering and Gamson (1987, p. 2) identified seven principles of good practice in undergraduate education, which

1. encourage contact between students and faculty,
2. develop reciprocity and cooperation among students,
3. encourage active learning,
4. give prompt feedback,
5. emphasize time on task,
6. communicate high expectations, and
7. respect diverse talents and ways of learning.

All of these principles should be considered when providing feedback to students in the clinical area. Certainly, providing "prompt feedback" is particularly relevant. If more time passes before you give feedback on learning experiences, then you will find it more difficult to remember details and provide effective feedback (Gaberson et al., 2015).

Including students' self-assessments when providing feedback is a critical element of the process. Throughout their careers, health-care professionals are encouraged to reflect on their own practice. This needed reflection can be developed by opening any feedback session with open-ended questions that invite learners to share their reflections and self-assessments. This strategy can soften perceptions of harshness associated with corrective feedback and bring unexpected questions and issues into the discussion (Ramani & Krackov, 2012).

All too often feedback is viewed as educator driven (Molloy et al., 2020), with instructors assuming primary responsibility for initiating and directing sessions. A more learner-centred approach encourages students to take a central role in the process and to seek opportunities to gather feedback from instructors and others in the practice area (Rudland et al., 2013).

A Strategy to Try ▶ *Beyond Just "Good Job" or "Needs Work"*
When offering feedback, try these five simple steps to go beyond just "good job" or "needs work."

1. *Affirm* positive aspects of what a student has done well.
2. *Explore* the student's own understanding of and feelings about the experience.
3. *Pick up on* any area that the student identifies as needing work.
4. *Identify* any additional areas where the student needs to improve, including an explanation of why these areas are important.
5. Provide an opportunity for the student to *reflect on and respond to* (in writing if possible) the feedback.

Grading

Grading, whether with a numerical value, letter grade, or pass/fail designation, indicates the degree of accomplishment achieved by a learner. Differentiating between *norm-referenced grading* and *criterion-referenced grading* is important. The former evaluates a student's performance compared with that of other students in a group or program, determining whether the performance is better than, worse than, or equivalent to that of other students (Gaberson et al., 2015). The latter evaluates a student's performance in relation to predetermined criteria and does not consider the performance of other students (Gaberson et al., 2015).

Criterion-referenced grading reflects only individual accomplishment. If all of the participants in a learning group demonstrate strong clinical skills, then they all earn top grades. In contrast, a learner's grade in norm-referenced grading reflects accomplishment in relation to others in the group. Only a select few can earn top grades, most will receive mid-level grades, and at least some will receive failing grades. Norm-referenced grading is based on the symmetrical statistical model of a bell or normal distribution curve.

The advantages of norm-referenced grading include the opportunity to compare students in a particular location with national norms, to highlight assignments that are too difficult or too easy, and to monitor grade distributions such as too many students receiving high or overinflated grades (Centre for the Study of Higher Education, 2002). The disadvantages of norm-referenced grading centre on the notion that one student's achievement, success, and even failure can depend unfairly on the performances of others. *Grade inflation*, an upward trend in grades awarded to students, has led many programs in the health disciplines to establish rigorous admission requirements and use a pass/fail grading approach.

Criterion-referenced grading judges student achievement against objective criteria outlined in course objectives and expected outcomes without consideration of what other students have or have not achieved. The process is transparent, and students can link their grades to their performance on predictable and set tasks (Centre for the Study of Higher Education, 2002). In turn, this approach can consider an individual student's learning needs and build in opportunities for remediation when needed (Winstrom, n.d.). One disadvantage of criterion-referenced grading is that instructors need more time for it. Also, awarding special recognition with prizes or scholarships to excelling students might not be as clear-cut when students are not compared with their peers.

A Strategy to Try ▶ *Can All Students Be above Average?*
Consider the advantages and disadvantages of evaluation approaches that are norm referenced (comparing students with other students) and criterion referenced (comparing students to set criteria). Discuss with your students when comparing their achievements with others in the group can be useful and when evaluating their performance only in relation to set criteria can be useful. How can clinical teachers incorporate ideas from both approaches into practice?

METHODS OF EVALUATING STUDENTS

Professional expectations dictate that all health-care practitioners must demonstrate prescribed proficiencies. Assessing, evaluating, providing feedback to, and ultimately assigning grades to students in clinical courses require teachers to implement a variety of evaluation methods. Going beyond measuring students' performance on standardized tests and check-lists is essential. Here we discuss methods of evaluating students that invite collaboration, tap into what students know, and identify future learning needs.

Instructor Observation

Instructor observation is one of the most commonly implemented methods of evaluating students. Instructor observation, also referred to as clinical performance assessment, provides important information about context-ual aspects of a learning situation (O'Connor, 2015). Knowing the context of why a student acted in a particular way can provide a more complete understanding of behaviour. If a task was not completed on time, knowing that the student reasoned that it was more important to stop and listen to clients' or patients' concerns can help instructors to make inferences about students' strengths and weaknesses. Yet anxiety about the experi-ence of being observed is well known to all of us. At what point is the stress of achieving course outcomes equivalent to the stress inherent in actual practice conditions? Does performance anxiety help or hinder evaluation?

Performance anxiety can be expected during instructor-observed activities (Cheung & Au, 2011; Weeks & Horan, 2013; Welsh, 2014). Instructional strategies that decrease performance anxiety include (1) demonstrating skills with supplemental sessions in laboratory settings before students complete skills in clinical settings and (2) arranging oppor-tunities for peers to observe and evaluate one another. Engaging students in non-evaluated discussion time can also help to reduce their anxiety (Melrose & Shapiro, 1999). Furthermore, inviting students to complete a self-assessment of any instructor-observed activity can help to make the experience collaborative.

Self-Assessment

Self-assessment opportunities can be made available and acknowledged to help students develop critical awareness and reflexivity (Dearnley & Meddings, 2007). Self-assessment is a necessary skill for lifelong learning (Boud, 1995). Practitioners in self-regulating health professions are required to self-assess. When students become familiar with the process during their education, they enter their professions with a stronger capacity for assessing and developing needed competencies (Kajander-Unkuri et al., 2013).

Self-assessment can shed light on the incidental, surprise, or unexpected learning (Chapter 3) that can occur beyond the intended goals and objectives of a clinical course. Pose questions such as "What surprised you when . . . ?" or "Can you talk about what happened that you didn't expect when . . . ?" Encouraging students to identify and then discuss their incidental learning in individual ways helps to build their confidence.

A cautionary note: self-assessments can be flawed. The most common flaw is that people often overrate themselves, indicating inaccurately that they are above average (Davis et al., 2006; Dunning et al., 2004; Mort & Hansen, 2010; Pisklakov et al., 2014). They might not accurately identify areas of weakness (Regehr & Eva, 2006) or overestimate their skills and performance (Baxter & Norman, 2011; Galbraith et al., 2008). Students who are the least competent in other areas of study are the least able to self-assess accurately (Austin & Gregory, 2007; Colthart et al., 2008). Balancing students' reflections on their activities with valid assessments of their progress and achievements is not straightforward (Melrose, 2017). Despite the flaws of self-assessment, inviting students to contribute their perceptions of what they have learned and what they still do not know is a critical aspect of evaluation.

Peer Assessment

Peer assessment, in which individuals of similar status evaluate the performance of their peers and provide feedback, can also help students to develop a critical attitude toward their own and others' practice (Laske, 2019; Mass et al., 2014; Sluijsmans et al., 2003). The advantages of peer assessment include opportunities for students to think more deeply about the activity being assessed, to gain insight into how others tackle similar problems, and to give and receive constructive criticism (Rush et al., 2012). The disadvantages include peers who have limited knowledge of a situation, show bias toward their friends, and hesitate to award low marks for poor work because they fear offending their peers (Rush et al., 2012). Personalities or learning styles might not be compatible among peers, and students might believe that they spend less individualized time with instructors when being reviewed by peers (Secomb, 2008). Instructors need to remain involved with any peer assessment activity in order to correct inaccurate or insufficient peer feedback (Hodgson et al., 2014).

Peer and self-assessments often differ from clinical teachers' assessments, indicating that neither of them can substitute for teacher assessment (Mehrdad et al., 2012). Even though peer assessments of students' clinical performance cannot be expected to provide a complete picture of students' strengths and areas needing improvement, they are a useful method of evaluation and should be incorporated whenever possible. When students step into the role of evaluator, either of themselves or of others at a similar stage of learning, they gain a new perspective on the teaching role. This familiarity might help them to believe that they are actively participating in the evaluation of themselves and others.

Anecdotal Notes

Anecdotal notes are the collections of information that instructors record, either by hand or electronically, to describe student performance in clinical practice (Hall, 2013). Notes are usually completed daily or weekly on all students and provide snapshots of their clients/patients and skills. Instructors are expected to complete anecdotal notes after observing a student complete a client/patient care procedure or report. Notes are also completed after incidents in which students have behaved in unusual or concerning ways, such as difficulty completing previously learned skills, showing poor decision making, appearing to be unprepared, or behaving in an unprofessional manner (Gardner & Suplee, 2010).

Each anecdotal note should be completed as soon as possible after observing a student's performance or concerning incident, and it should only address that one performance or incident. Each note should include a description of the client/patient and the required skills as well as objective observations of the student's behaviour actually seen and heard by the instructor. Individual anecdotal notes are narrative accounts of an experience at one point in time and should be shared with students (Gaberson et al., 2015; O'Connor, 2015). Many instructors invite students to respond or add to anecdotal notes after students review and reflect on them.

Cumulatively, individual anecdotal notes can be reviewed over time for patterns of behaviour useful in evaluating student progress and continued learning needs. These notes should be retained after courses end since disputes over clinical grades might occur (Heaslip & Scammel, 2012). Anecdotal notes need not just be descriptions of students' behaviour. They can and should also include the specific suggestions and guidance that teachers provide to support their students in being successful.

Records of students' assignments should also be retained. These records can reflect how different opportunities were available to students to demonstrate required skills. They can illustrate the situations in which students performed well and poorly. These records have also been used to defend instructors' decisions to fail students who assert that they were given overly difficult assignments (O'Connor, 2015).

A Strategy to Try ▶ *Balancing Instructor, Student, and Peer Assessments*
Imagine creating three piles of documentation for each student in a clinical course. The first pile contains instructors' observations and anecdotal notes. The second pile contains students' self-assessments and responses to instructors' anecdotal notes. The third pile contains peer assessments of students' work. Are the piles balanced and equal? Should they be? Which, if any, additional opportunities could be built into your teaching practice to balance instructor, peer, and self-assessments?

LEARNING CONTRACTS

Adult educator Malcolm Knowles (1975, p. 130) explains that a learning contract is a "means of reconciling the 'imposed' requirements from institutions and society with the learners' need to be self-directing. It enables them to blend these requirements in with their own personal goals and objectives, to choose ways of achieving them and the measure of their own progress toward achieving them." In other words, the goal of any learning contract is to promote learner self-direction, autonomy, and independence. As Knowles emphasizes, learning contracts must include what is to be learned, how it will be learned, and how that learning will be evaluated.

As part of continuing competence requirements, most health-care professionals are expected to engage in self-directed learning activities. These activities demonstrate to regulatory bodies that these professionals can identify what they need to know, how they will learn it, and how they will evaluate their learning. Initiating learning contracts with students can help to prepare them for this practice requirement.

Traditionally, learning contracts have been used mainly with students who are struggling to meet clinical objectives and standards or whose performance is perceived as unsafe (Frank & Scharff, 2013; Gregory et al., 2009). In these instances, instructors must clearly identify the outcomes to be addressed and work collaboratively with students to determine the resources and assistance needed to address the issues (Atherton, 2013). A contract must be signed by both instructor and student, and both must document the progress made or not made after each clinical experience.

Extending the idea of learning contracts beyond struggling students is becoming more common. Learning contracts can be a teaching strategy that fosters motivation and independent learning in students in nursing (Chan & Wai-tong, 2000; Timmins, 2002), respiratory care (Rye, 2008), physiotherapy (Ramli et al., 2013), and clinical psychology (Keary & Byrne, 2013). Although incorporating learning contracts for all students and not just those who struggle might initially seem to be time consuming, the result can be rewarding.

A Strategy to Try ▶ *Model Self-Direction in a Learning Contract*
Model the kind of self-direction that professionals need in everyday practice by creating your own learning contract. Think about one of your own learning needs. Write down what you need to learn, how you will learn it, and how you will evaluate the learning.

Keep the learning need simple, manageable, and easy to understand. If your regulatory body requires you to use learning contracts or a similar process, then use the language and protocols required by your profession. Share your contract with students early in the course, and encourage them to support and critique your progress. If you are not comfortable with sharing your own learning contract, then create one that illustrates how a member of your professional group might learn.

FAILURE

Despite clear objectives, thoughtful teaching strategies, and a supportive learning environment, some learners simply are not able to demonstrate the competencies required to pass a clinical course. The experience of failure can be devastating for all involved (Black et al., 2014; Handwerker, 2018; Larocque & Luhanga, 2013).

The accepted norm within clinical teaching is that, at the beginning of any educational event, participants will be thoroughly informed about both the learning outcomes that they are expected to achieve and specific institutional policies that apply when those objectives are not met. Similarly, learners must be informed promptly when an evaluator begins to notice problems with their progress. Typically, learners are informed of problems through collaborative formative evaluations and feedback long before a final failing summative evaluation.

The daily anecdotal notes or records of learners' actions mentioned above are essential throughout any evaluative process, but they become particularly important when a learner is in danger of failing. Most formative or mid-term evaluation instruments are designed to provide feedback on learning progress and identify further work needed. Summative or final evaluations describe the extent to which learners have achieved course objectives. Thus, when a learner is not progressing satisfactorily, a prompt, documented learning contract or plan can be invaluable in identifying specific behaviours that the instructor and student agree to work on together. Instructors' supervisors must be informed about any students who are struggling or unsafe, and they must be kept up to date throughout the process.

In some cases, learners might choose not to collaborate on a remedial learning contract or plan. Documenting students' and instructors' perceptions of this process is important as well. Providing students with information about institutional procedures for withdrawing from the learning event or appealing a final assessment is essential in demonstrating an open, fair, and transparent process of evaluation.

Given the emotional nature of clinical failure, those involved in the process might not be able to identify immediately how the experience is one of positive growth and learning. In fact, having opportunities to talk and debrief can help both students and instructors. For university, college, and technical institute students, counselling services are generally available through the institution. For instructors, both full-time continuing faculty and those employed on a contract or sessional basis, counselling services might be available from an employee assistance program.

Knowing that students might fail and that counselling services might help, you can distribute pamphlets outlining contact information for those counselling services to all students in the group at the beginning of the course. If the information is already at hand, then referring an individual learner to the service when needed normalizes the suggestion. In some cases, without compromising confidentiality, actually accompanying an individual to a counselling appointment or walking with the person into the counselling services area can begin to ease the devastation.

Clinical instructors and preceptors can be reluctant to fail students. The phrase "failure to fail" (Duffy, 2003, 2004) is used to describe a growing trend toward passing students who do not meet course objectives and outcomes. In one study, "37% of mentors [preceptors] passed student nurses, despite concerns about competencies or attitude, or who felt they should fail" (Gainsbury, 2010, p.1).

One key reason that clinical instructors fail to fail is lack of support (Black et al., 2014; Bush et al., 2013; Duffy, 2004; Gainsbury, 2010; Larocque & Luhanga, 2013). When universities overturn decisions to fail on appeal and require detailed written evidence justifying an instructor's decision to fail a student, clinical instructors can feel as though they are not supported (Gainsbury, 2010). As caring health professionals, instructors can believe that failing is an uncaring action (Scanlan et al., 2001). Many also fear that a student's failure will reflect badly on them and that others will judge them as bad teachers (Gainsbury, 2010).

However, health-care professionals have a duty of care to protect the public from harm. When students whose practice is unsafe and who fail to meet required course outcomes are not assigned failing grades, instructors must question whether they are neglecting their duty of care (Black et al., 2014). The reputation of the professional program can be diminished as a result of failing to fail a student (Larocque & Luhanga, 2013). Viewing clinical failure in a positive light is difficult for both students and instructors. Learning from the experience is what counts. As Samuel Beckett wrote, "Ever tried. Ever failed. No matter. Try again. Fail again. Fail better" (1983, p. 11).

A Strategy to Try ▶ *Fail Better*
How can clinical instructors follow Beckett's sage advice and "fail better"? To begin, have a clear working knowledge of course outcomes. Next maintain detailed documentation that gives an objective and balanced picture of student behaviours and agreed-upon strategies for improving them. Connect with any available support services for students and for instructors. Finally, consider the implications of failing to fail.

METHODS OF EVALUATING TEACHING

Clinical programs in the health professions usually stipulate specific assessment tools to be used to evaluate clinical teachers. Commonly, students are given anonymous questionnaires to complete at the ends of their courses, and supervisors complete standardized performance appraisals. Clinical instructors employed as full-time continuing faculty members might be involved in constructing these tools, but sessional instructors or those employed on a contract basis are seldom consulted. Although clinical instructors might have little control over the tools of evaluation required by their programs, performance appraisal documents are likely to include opportunities for self-assessments, which can be framed as teaching portfolios. Collecting information from a variety of assessment tools over a period of time is necessary to construct accurate student evaluations, and the same is true for instructor evaluation (Billings & Halstead, 2012).

Teaching portfolios, also called teaching dossiers or teaching profiles, are pieces of evidence collected over time and used to highlight teaching strengths and accomplishments (Barrett, n.d.; Edgerton et al., 2002; Seldin, 1997; Shulman, 1998). The collection of evidence can be paper based or electronic. Teaching portfolios can usually be integrated into self-assessment sections of performance appraisal requirements. No two teaching portfolios are alike, and the content pieces can be arranged in creative and unique ways.

Portfolios usually begin with an explanation of the instructor's teaching philosophy. In Chapter 2, we provided suggestions for crafting a personal teaching philosophy statement. When the purpose of a portfolio is to contribute self-assessment information to performance appraisals, goals should also be explained. Reflective inquiry is a critical element of any portfolio, and reflections on teaching approaches that failed, as well as those that succeeded, should be included (Lyons, 2006). Both goals that have been accomplished and specific plans for accomplishing future goals should be noted. Since clinical teachers must maintain competencies in both their clinical practice and their teaching practice, another segment of the portfolio could list certifications earned; workshops, conferences, or other educational events attended; papers written about clinical teaching in a course; and awards received.

Teaching products could constitute another segment, such as writing a case study about a typical client or patient in your practice setting, developing a student orientation module for your students, crafting a student learning activity such as a game or puzzle, devising an innovative strategy to support a struggling student, or demonstrating a skill on video. Mementoes such as thank-you messages from students, colleagues, agency staff, or clients/patients could also be included. Distinguish between content that can be made public and that which should be kept private. For example, a student learning activity might be made public by publishing it in a journal article or on a teaching website, whereas mementoes would be private and likely shared only with supervisors.

If your program does not provide students with an opportunity to offer formative evaluation to instructors of how the course is going, create this opportunity for them. Rather than waiting for student feedback at the end of the course, seek it at mid-term. Provide a mechanism that is fully anonymous, for example an online survey, in which students can comment on what is going well, what is not going well, and what advice they would like to give to the instructor. In your portfolio, discuss this formative feedback, your responses to it, and your evaluation of the process.

As the above examples illustrate, the possibilities for demonstrating instructional achievements are limitless. Each item in your portfolio should include a brief statement explaining why it is included and how it reflects a valid and authentic assessment of teaching achievements (Barrett, n.d.). Two other pieces of content commonly included in teaching portfolios are responses from student questionnaires and peer assessments.

Students' assessments of their instructors' teaching effectiveness are most often collected through anonymous questionnaires at the end of the course. Anonymity is important since students can fear that rating their instructor poorly could affect their grades. Completing the questionnaire is optional, and instructors must not be involved in administering or collecting the questionnaires (Center for Teaching and Learning, n.d.).

Research indicates that instructors are more likely to receive higher ratings from students who are highly motivated and interested in the course content (Benton & Cashin, 2012). Although students' ratings of their instructors yield valuable interpretations of instructors' engagement of students and enthusiasm, students are not subject matter experts and therefore cannot evaluate the accuracy and depth of instructors' knowledge (Oermann, 2015). In general, college students' ratings of their instructors tend to be more statistically reliable, valid, and relatively free from bias than any other data used for instructor evaluation. They are only one source of data, however, and should be used in combination with other sources of information (Benton & Cashin, 2012). Including samples of responses from student questionnaires is expected in most teaching portfolios.

If peer assessments of instructors are not usually part of your program, then consider including them in your teaching portfolio. Acquire permission for peer assessment from both program and clinical site administrators. Peer observers can be other teachers in the program or staff at the clinical agency, and they should be provided with an evaluation instrument. For example, Chickering and Gamson's (1987) seven principles can guide peer observers in framing their feedback. Introduce the peer observer to students in the group and relevant agency staff members. Ensure that students understand that the purpose of the observation is instructor evaluation, not student evaluation (Center for Teaching and Learning, n.d.).

A Strategy to Try ▶ *What's in Your Teaching Portfolio?*

If you have not done so already, initiate a teaching portfolio, and keep adding to it throughout your teaching career. Visualize a large artist's case that holds all of the items that an artist would use to illustrate or sell works. For example, a portrait painter's case might contain a black-and-white sketch of a young girl, a full-colour family portrait, and a detailed replica of a classic piece. Each item would have personal relevance to the artist and reflect their skills. Similarly, your teaching portfolio should contain items that illustrate your individual interests and expertise. What's in *your* teaching portfolio?

CONCLUSION

Evaluating our students and ourselves is a critical aspect of clinical teaching. In this chapter, we discussed methods of evaluating students and methods of evaluating teachers. The process of evaluating students requires clinical teachers to make judgments about whether students are meeting objectives or not based on information gathered and recorded throughout the course. Clinical teachers measure attributes of learning with standardized instruments and assess learning through inferences about how students are applying theory to practice based on observations in different situations.

Meaningful evaluation goes beyond identifying students' progress in relation to course objectives and outcomes. Deep learning occurs when teachers provide their students with specific and individualized feedback. Students' self-assessments of their strengths and plans for improvement should frame any feedback conversation. Ultimately, instructors must assign grades. They can be determined through a norm-referenced approach that compares students with other students or through a criterion-referenced approach that compares students to set criteria.

Clinical teachers can evaluate students using instructors' observations, students' self-assessments, and peer assessments. Daily anecdotal notes should be kept and shared with students, recording instructors' objective observations of their clinical performance. Learning contracts can be co-created with all students, though traditionally they have been used mainly with students whose practice is unsafe or who are not meeting course objectives.

Student failure is a devastating experience. All too often clinical teachers and preceptors fail to fail students whose practice is unsafe or who have not met course outcomes. Evaluating students requires that those involved consider the duty of care for all health professionals to protect the public from harm.

We also discussed methods of evaluating our own teaching. We suggested creating a teaching portfolio as a method of self-assessment. Teaching portfolios can include statements of personal teaching philosophy, responses from student questionnaires, and peer assessments. They can showcase a variety of achievements and reflections.

REFERENCES

Archer, J. (2010). State of the science in health profession education: Effective feedback. *Medical Education, 44*(1), 101–108. https://doi.org/10.1111/j.1365-2923.2009.03546.x

Assessment. (n.d.). In *The glossary of education reform*. http://edglossary.org/

Atherton, J. (2013). *Learning and teaching: Learning contracts* [Fact sheet]. http://www.learningandteaching.info/teaching/learning_contracts.htm

Austin, Z., & Gregory, p. (2007). Evaluating the accuracy of pharmacy students' self-assessment skills. *American Journal of Pharmaceutical Education, 71*(5), 1–8.

Barrett, H. (n.d.). *Dr. Helen Barrett's electronic portfolios* [Website]. http://electronicportfolios.com/

Baxter, P., & Norman, G. (2011). Self-assessment or self-deception? A negative association between self-assessment and performance. *Journal of Advanced Nursing, 67*(11), 2406–2413. https://doi.org/10.1111/j.1365-2648.2011.05658.x

Beckett, S. (1983). *Worstward ho*. Grove Press.

Benton, S., & Cashin, W. (2012). *Student ratings of teaching: A summary of research and literature*. Idea Paper 50. The Idea Centre. http://www.ntid.rit.edu/sites/default/files/academic_affairs/Sumry%20of%20Res%20%2350%20Benton%202012.pdf

Billings, D., & Halstead, J. (2012). *Teaching in nursing: A guide for faculty* (4th ed.). Elsevier.

Black, S., Curzio, J., & Terry, L. (2014). Failing a student nurse: A new horizon of moral courage. *Nursing Ethics, 21*(2), 224–238.

Boud, D. (1995). *Enhancing learning through self-assessment*. Kogan Page.

Bradshaw, M., & Lowenstein, A. (2014). *Innovative teaching strategies in nursing and related health professions education* (6th ed.). Jones & Bartlett.

Brookhart, S. (2008). *How to give effective feedback to your students*. Association for Supervision and Curriculum Development.

Bush, H., Schreiber, R., & Oliver, S. (2013). Failing to fail: Clinicians' experience of assessing underperforming dental students. *European Journal of Dental Education, 17*(4), 198–207. https://doi.org/10.1111/eje.12036

Carless, D., & Boud, D. (2018). The development of student feedback literacy: Enabling uptake of feedback. *Assessment & Evaluation in Higher Education, 43*(8), 1315–1325. https://doi.org/10.1080/02602938.2018.1463354

Carnegie Mellon. (n.d.) *What is the difference between formative and summative assessment?* [Fact sheet]. Eberly Center for Teaching Excellence, Carnegie Mellon University, Pittsburgh, PA. http://www.cmu.edu/teaching/assessment/basics/formative-summative.html

Center for Teaching and Learning. (n.d.). *Peer observation guidelines and recommendations* [Fact sheet]. University of Minnesota, Minneapolis, MN. http://www1.umn.edu/ohr/teachlearn/resources/peer/guidelines/index.html

Centre for the Study of Higher Education. (2002). *A comparison of norm-referencing and criterion-referencing methods for determining student grades in higher education.* Australian Universities Teaching Committee. http://www.cshe.unimelb.edu.au/assessinglearning/06/normvcrit6.html

Chan, S., & Wai-tong, C. (2000). Implementing contract learning in a clinical context: Report on a study. *Journal of Advanced Nursing, 31*(2), 298–305.

Cheung, R., & Au, T. (2011). Nursing students' anxiety and clinical performance. *Journal of Nursing Education, 50*(5), 286–289. https://doi.org/10.3928/01484834-20110131-08

Chickering, A., & Gamson, Z. (1987). Seven principles for good practice in undergraduate education. *American Association for Higher Education AAHE Bulletin, 39*(7), 2–6.

Colthart, I., Bagnall, G., Evans, A., Allbutt, H., Haig, A., Illing, J., & McKinstry, B. (2008). The effectiveness of self-assessment on the identification of learning needs, learner activity, and impact on clinical practice: BEME Guide No. 10. *Medical Teacher, 30,* 124–145.

Concordia University. (n.d.) *How to provide feedback to health professions students* [Wiki]. http://www.wikihow.com/Provide-Feedback-to-Health-Professions-Students

Davis, D., Mazmanian, P., Fordis, M., Van Harrison, R., Thorpe, K., & Perrier, L. (2006). Accuracy of physician self-assessment compared with observed measures of competence: A systematic review. *The Journal of the American Medical Association, 296*(9), 1094–1102.

Dearnley, C., & Meddings, F. (2007). Student self-assessment and its impact on learning: A pilot study. *Nurse Education Today, 27*(4), 333–340.

Duffy, K. (2003). *Failing students: A qualitative study of factors that influence the decisions regarding assessment of students' competence in practice.* Glasgow Caledonian Nursing and Midwifery Research Centre. http://www.nmc-uk.org/Documents/Archived%20Publications/1Research%20papers/Kathleen_Duffy_Failing_Students2003.pdf

Duffy, K. (2004). Mentors need more support to fail incompetent students. *British Journal of Nursing, 13*(10), 582. https://doi.org/10.12968/bjon.2004.13.10.13042

Dunning, D., Heath, C., & Suls, J. (2004). Flawed self-assessment: Implications for health education and the workplace. *Psychological Science in the Public Interest,*

5(3), 69–106. https://faculty-gsb.stanford.edu/heath/documents/PSPI%20-%20Biased%20Self%20Views.pdf

Edgerton, R., Hutching, P., & Quinlan, K. (2002). *The teaching portfolio: Capturing the scholarship of teaching*. American Association of Higher Education.

Emerson, R. (2007). *Nursing education in the clinical setting*. Mosby.

Frank, T., & Scharff, L. (2013). Learning contracts in undergraduate courses: Impacts on student behaviors and academic performance. *Journal of the Scholarship of Teaching and Learning, 13*(4), 36–53.

Gaberson, K., Oermann, M., & Shellenbarger, T. (2015). *Clinical teaching strategies in nursing* (4th ed.). Springer.

Gainsbury, S. (2010). Mentors passing students despite doubts over ability. *Nursing Times, 106*(16), 1–3.

Galbraith, R., Hawkins, R., & Holmboe, E. (2008). Making self-assessment more effective. *Journal of Continuing Education in the Health Professions, 28*(1), 20–24.

Gardner, M., & Suplee, p. (2010). *Handbook of clinical teaching in nursing and health sciences*. Jones & Bartlett.

Gregory, D., Guse, L., Dick, D., Davis, P., & Russell, C. (2009). What clinical learning contracts reveal about nursing education and patient safety. *Canadian Nurse, 105*(8), 20–25.

Hall, M. (2013). An expanded look at evaluating clinical performance: Faculty use of anecdotal notes in the US and Canada. *Nurse Education in Practice, 13*, 271–276.

Handwerker, S. (2018). Challenges experienced by nursing students overcoming one course failure: A phenomenological research study. *Teaching and Learning in Nursing, 13*, 168–173.

Heaslip, V., & Scammel, J. (2012). Failing underperforming students: The role of grading in practice assessment. *Nursing Education in Practice, 12*(2), 95–100.

Hodgson, P., Chan, K., & Liu, J. (2014). Outcomes of synergetic peer assessment: First-year experience. *Assessment and Evaluation in Higher Education, 39*(2), 168–179.

Kajander-Unkuri, S., Meretoja, R., Katajisto, J., Saarikoski, M., Salminen, L., Suhonene, R., & Leino-Kilpi, H. (2013). Self-assessed level of competence of graduating nursing students and factors related to it. *Nurse Education Today, 34*(5), 795–801.

Keary, E., & Byrne, M. (2013). A trainee's guide to managing clinical placements. *The Irish Psychologist, 39*(4), 104–110.

Knowles, M. (1975). *Self-directed learning*. Association Press.

Larocque, S., & Luhanga, F. (2013). Exploring the issue of failure to fail in a nursing program. *International Journal of Nursing Education Scholarship, 10*(1), 1–8.

Laske, R. (2019). Peer evaluation of clinical teaching practices. *Teaching and Learning in Nursing, 14*(1), 65–68.

Lyons, N. (2006). Reflective engagement as professional development in the lives of university teachers. *Teachers and Teaching: Theory and Practice, 12*(2), 151–168.

Marsh, S., Cooper, K., Jordan, G., Merrett, S., Scammell, J., & Clark, V. (2005). *Assessment of students in health and social care: Managing failing students in practice*. Bournemouth University Publishing.

Mass, M., Sluijsmans, D., van der Wees, P., Heerkens, Y., Nijhuis-van der Sanden, M., & van der Vleuten, C. (2014). Why peer assessment helps to improve clinical performance in undergraduate physical therapy education: A mixed methods design. *BMC Medical Education, 14*, 117. https://doi.org/10.1186/1472-6920-14-117

Mehrdad, N., Bigdeli, S., & Ebrahimi, H. (2012). A comparative study on self, peer and teacher evaluation to evaluate clinical skills of nursing students. *Procedia– Social and Behavioral Science, 47*, 1847–1852.

Melrose, S. (2017). Balancing reflection and validity in health profession students' self-assessment. *International Journal of Learning, Teaching and Educational Research, 16*(8), 65–76.

Melrose, S., & Shapiro, B. (1999). Students' perceptions of their psychiatric mental health clinical nursing experience: A personal construct theory explanation. *Journal of Advanced Nursing, 30*(6), 1451–1458.

Molloy, E., Ajjawi, R., Bearman, M., Noble, C., Rudland, J., & Ryan, A. (2020). Challenging feedback myths: Values, learner involvement and promoting effects beyond the immediate task. *Medical Education, 54*(1), 33–39. https://doi.org/10.1111/medu.13802

Mort, J., & Hansen, D. (2010). First-year pharmacy students' self-assessment of communication skills and the impact of video review. *American Journal of Pharmaceutical Education, 74*(5), 1–7.

O'Connor, A. (2015). *Clinical instruction and evaluation.* Jones & Bartlett.

Oermann, M. (2015). *Teaching in nursing and role of the educator.* Springer.

Pisklakov, S., Rimal, J., & McGuirt, S. (2014). Role of self-evaluation and self-assessment in medical student and resident education. *British Journal of Education, Society and Behavioral Science, 4*(1), 1–9.

Ramani, S., & Krackov, S. (2012). Twelve tips for giving feedback effectively in the clinical environment. *Medical Teacher, 34*, 787–791.

Ramli, A., Joseph, L., & Lee, S. (2013). Learning pathways during clinical placement of physiotherapy students: A Malaysian experience of using learning contracts and reflective diaries. *Journal of Educational Evaluation in the Health Professions, 10*, 6. https://doi.org/10.3352/jeehp.2013.10.6

Ramsden, p. (1992). *Learning to teach in higher education.* Routledge.

Regehr, G., & Eva, K. (2006). Self-assessment, self-direction, and the self-regulating professional. *Clinical Orthopaedics and Related Research, 449*, 34–38. http://innovationlabs.com/r3p_public/rtr3/pre/pre-read/Self-assessment.Regher.Eva.2006.pdf

Rudland, J., Wilkinson, T., Wearn, A., Nicol, P., Tunny, T., Owen, C., & O'Keefe, M. (2013). A student-centred model for educators. *The Clinical Teacher, 10*(2), 92–102.

Rush, S., Firth, T., Burke, L., & Marks-Maran, D. (2012). Implementation and evaluation of peer assessment of clinical skills for first year student nurses. *Nurse Education in Practice, 12*(4), 2219–2226.

Rye, K. (2008). Perceived benefits of the use of learning contracts to guide clinical education in respiratory care students. *Respiratory Care, 53*(11), 1475–1481.

Scales, D. E. (1943). Differences between measurement criteria of pure scientists and of classroom teachers. *Journal of Educational Research 37,* 1–13.

Scanlan, J., Care, D., & Glessler, S. (2001). Dealing with the unsafe student in clinical practice. *Nurse Educator, 26*(1), 23–27.

Secomb, J. (2008). A systematic review of peer teaching and learning in clinical education. *Journal of Clinical Nursing, 17*(6), 703–716. https://doi.org/10.1111/j.1365-2702.2007.01954.x

Seldin, p. (1997). *The teaching portfolio: A practical guide to improved performance and promotion/tenure decisions* (2nd ed.). Anker.

Shulman, L. (1998). Teacher portfolios: A theoretical activity. In N. Lyons (Ed.), *With portfolio in hand: Validating the new teacher professionalism* (pp. 23–37). Teachers College Press.

Sluijsmans, D., Van Merriënboer, J., Brand-Gruwel, S., & Bastiaens, T. (2003). The training of peer assessment skills to promote the development of reflection skills in teacher education. *Studies in Education Evaluation, 29,* 23–42.

Timmins, F. (2002). The usefulness of learning contracts in nurse education: The Irish perspective. *Nurse Education in Practice, 2*(3), 190–196. https://doi.org/10.1054/nepr.2002.0069

Walsh, T., Jairath, N., Paterson, M., & Grandjean, C. (2010). Quality and safety education for nurses clinical evaluation tool. *Journal of Nursing Education, 49*(9), 517–522.

Weeks, B., & Horan, S. (2013). A video-based learning activity is effective for preparing physiotherapy students for practical examinations. *Physiotherapy, 99,* 292–297.

Welsh, p. (2014). How first year occupational therapy students rate the degree to which anxiety negatively impacts on their performance in skills assessments: A pilot study at the University of South Australia. *Ergo, 3*(2), 31–38. http://www.ojs.unisa.edu.au/index.php/ergo/article/view/927

Winstrom, E. (n.d.). *Norm-referenced or criterion-referenced? You be the judge!* [Fact sheet]. http://www.brighthubeducation.com/student-assessment-tools/72677-norm-referenced-versus-criterion-referenced-assessments/?cid=parsely_rec

8

Preceptors

Essential to Learner Success

While we teach, we learn.
SENECA THE YOUNGER (N.D., BOOK I, LETTER 7, SEC. 8)

Precepting is an organized, evidence-based, outcome-driven approach to assuring competent practice (Eley, 2015). Clinical health education often employs a preceptor model for senior practicum courses and frequently as part of orienting new employees. Through clinical experiences and orientation activities, learners acquire knowledge and essential skills for professional practice. The preceptor plays a vital role in developing students as professionals and a critical role in successfully integrating new staff.

For student learners, a representative from the student's institution is often part of the teaching-learning team along with the student and a preceptor who is an employee of the clinical agency. Each member of the trio usually has specific roles and responsibilities, with the faculty representative often supporting and advising the preceptor. Although the preceptor has important roles in student evaluation, the faculty member usually makes critical decisions on final grades and whether a learner passes or fails a practicum.

Being a preceptor for a student or new employee is an essential role but not one for which most preceptors are formally prepared. The short- and long-term success of the student or employee can be enhanced greatly by an excellent preceptor or affected negatively by a preceptor who is not well prepared for the role. Our goal in this chapter is to provide readers with knowledge, skills, and attitudes that are key to being an effective preceptor in the clinical setting. As with most careers, when you are well prepared and able to excel in a role, those with whom you work are positively affected. As you carry out your role well, your level of satisfaction with it is also enhanced. This leads to a positive cycle with affirmative effects on all involved, including recipients of care.

In this chapter, we discuss the difference between preceptoring and mentoring, examine the theoretical foundations of effective preceptoring, and present strategies for becoming and remaining a successful preceptor. We conclude with a discussion of the preceptor-preceptee relationship. The strategies included provide a road map for practitioners who are new to precepting. The chapter is infused with practical creative ideas and founded on theory, making it both a stand-alone chapter for educators embarking on being a great preceptor and part of the greater understanding of becoming skilled as a clinical educator.

THE DIFFERENCE BETWEEN A MENTOR AND A PRECEPTOR

The origin of the concept of *mentorship* is well documented. In Homer's *Odyssey*, a mentor, a wise and trusted friend of Odysseus, takes on the rearing of his son in his absence (Roberts, 1999). The mentor is depicted as an older, wiser male who takes on the responsibility for a younger male's learning and development, acting rather like a guardian. The term "mentor" is traditionally associated with professions such as medicine, law, and business, but it began appearing in nursing literature in the 1990s (Andrews & Wallis, 1999).

Much of the current literature on mentoring focuses on defining the concept, yet a precise and complete definition that is universally embraced remains elusive (Dawson, 2014; Gopee, 2011; Mentoring Resources, n.d.). To confuse it further, terms such as "preceptor," "coach," and "facilitator" are used interchangeably in some instances. In jurisdictions such as Great Britain, practising nurses who are responsible for students in the clinical area are called mentors, whereas in most North American jurisdictions these supervising nurses are called preceptors. Commonly, the term "mentor" is reserved for a longer-term personal development relationship between a less experienced person and a more experienced person, with the focus of the relationship on assistance, befriending, guiding, and advising (Eby et al., 2007). More concisely, the mentor is less focused on assessment and supervision and more focused on the mentee's well-being and career advancement (Eby et al., 2007).

In contrast, a preceptor-preceptee relationship is usually shorter term, and the preceptor has responsibility for teaching and assessing clinical performance. In the base definition of preceptor, the focus of the preceptor's work is on upholding a *precept* or law or tradition. Myrick and Yonge (2005, p. 4) define a nursing preceptor as a skilled practitioner who oversees students in a clinical setting to facilitate practical experience with patients.

The roles of mentor and preceptor do overlap. For example, a preceptor who has no concern for the well-being of the preceptee is not likely to provide the learner with a positive clinical experience. Likewise, a mentor who does not assess student practice will not have the information needed to be an effective mentor. The assessment in which a mentor engages is more likely to be formative and focused on providing the mentor with knowledge to fulfill the role of guide effectively.

Students in practice-based health-care professions rely on others to support, teach, and supervise them in practice settings. The underlying rationale for this approach to learning is the belief that working alongside practitioners aids students to become safe caregivers who are successfully socialized to the clinical world (Benner, 1984). In this chapter, we focus on the role of the preceptor.

THEORETICAL FOUNDATIONS OF EFFECTIVE PRECEPTORING

Effective preceptoring of students in health-care clinical environments can be understood by briefly examining adult learning theory, transformational learning theory, and the From Novice to Expert model. We will outline each theory or model and discuss it in relation to the preceptoring literature.

Adult Learning Theory

As described in Chapter 1, Malcolm Knowles (1984) is credited with naming the theory of andragogy in relation to adult learning. Andragogy emphasizes how adult learners differ from child learners in being self-directed and taking responsibility for their learning decisions. Furthermore, according to Knowles, adults want to know why they are learning something, need to learn experientially (including having the opportunity to make mistakes), use problem solving to learn, and learn most effectively if they can apply what they learn immediately. Knowles states that adults learn best if their teacher is primarily a facilitator or resource person. Smith (2002) discusses Knowles's theory, highlighting the ideas that learners move from being dependent to self-directed, accumulate a reservoir of experience and knowledge, and are internally motivated to learn. Given these principles of adult learning, teaching strategies such as simulations, role-playing, and case studies are considered useful. Likewise, clinical practicum learning opportunities with the student working alongside a preceptor are compatible with the principles of andragogy. Practicum students are directed by a more knowledgeable person (the preceptor) until they can accumulate experience and knowledge to be independent practitioners.

Sandlin et al. (2013) further our understanding of Knowles's theory with additional focus on his beliefs that adult learners are autonomous, rational, and capable of action and on the assumption that autonomy and rationality are desirable and attainable in adult learners. Their perspective on Knowles's fundamental views provides an interesting contrast in considering the role of preceptor in the clinical environment. The tenets of Knowles's adult learning theory offer no substantive role for the preceptors who hold responsibility for overseeing, guiding, and evaluating the work of the preceptee, for learners are thought to be totally autonomous and capable of independence. In contrast, as Sandlin et al. propose, adult learners might actually be at various levels of autonomy and rationality, and thus a skilled preceptor does have a role in adult learning.

Transformational Learning Theory

As explained in Chapter 1, Jack Mezirow (1995) is credited with making significant contributions to the theory of transformative learning. The essence of this theory is that learners must engage in critical reflection on their experiences in order to transform their beliefs, attitudes, and perspectives, which Mezirow terms their "meaning schemes." Others have critiqued some of his assumptions and views. Boyd and Myers (1988) note that learners must be open to changing their meaning schemes; to adopt new perspectives, they must realize that their old perspectives are no longer relevant. Dirkx et al. (2006, p. 123) emphasize the self-actualization possibilities of transformative learning with the statement that "learning is life—not a preparation for it." They note the importance of a relationship between the learner and others, which is required to make sense of one's perspective and to become aware of (and transform to) new meanings.

For Mezirow, the essence of learning is change. To be truly transformational, learners must engage in inquiry, critical thinking, and interaction with others. Brookfield (2000) adds that transformative learning must include a fundamental questioning of one's thoughts and actions. Reflection alone does not result in transformative learning unless this reflection includes an analysis of taken-for-granted assumptions.

The entry-to-practice competencies for health-care professionals include elements of critical reflection; adoption of professional values, beliefs, and attitudes; and ongoing questioning of taken-for-granted assumptions and values. If Mezirow is correct that acquiring a competency does require the involvement of others, then this becomes part of the role of the skilled preceptor. Preceptors might be well placed to encourage honest self-review and critical reflection that ends in learner transformation. In this view, preceptors need to be aware of strategies to engage learners in reflection, causing them to gaze deeply into long- and deeply held values and biases that they might not even be aware they hold.

The From Novice to Expert Model

Benner's (1984) well-used and much-respected From Novice to Expert model has implications for understanding the role of an effective preceptor for health-care learners. Although Benner focused on nursing students in the clinical setting, her theory likely applies to learners in other health-care disciplines. This model holds that nurses develop skills over time from both education (including clinical experience) and personal experience. The model identifies five levels of nursing experience: novice, advanced beginner, competent, proficient, and expert. Novices are beginners with no experience—they learn rule-governed tasks by following instructions. Advanced beginners have gained experience in actual nursing situations and recognize recurring elements that create principles that they can use to guide actions. Competent nurses have more clinical experience and use it to become more efficient in providing care. Proficient nurses have an understanding of the bigger picture that improves decision making and allows for changes in plans as needed. Experts no longer need principles or rules to guide actions—they use intuition to guide their flexible, highly proficient clinical approaches. As learners transition from novice to expert, they rely less on principles, they see a situation more holistically, and they engage in situations from the inside rather than the outside.

Preceptors can play a vital role in this transition. Benner's (1984) model requires clinical experience for the transition to occur, and guidance in the clinical situation is essential for successful transition. Preceptors need to have awareness of the needs of learners at various stages of the continuum and be attuned to the stage(s) at which their students are functioning. For example, a novice student needs a preceptor who provides more direct guidance in learning the rules to guide her or his actions. A preceptor for advanced beginners helps them to recognize recurring patterns and develop them into principles of effective care.

Benner (1984) also comments that expert clinicians might not be the most effective in preceptoring roles. They might have difficulty explaining their actions in a step-by-step manner because they function by intuition and might not be consciously aware of the rules and principles that they use to make clinical judgments. Analogous to riding a bike, beginners are aware of the steps needed to balance the bike, propel it forward, stop it, and avoid obstacles. An expert cyclist is able to ride without thinking about how to ride and thus might have a challenge in teaching a new cyclist.

STRATEGIES FOR BEING AND BECOMING A SUCCESSFUL PRECEPTOR

In this section, we focus on strategies for being (and becoming) a successful preceptor for students in various health-care professions in clinical learning environments. We also address the challenges and rewards of being a preceptor and the characteristics of effective preceptors. Our goal is to provide both new and established preceptors with new knowledge that can be used as a road map to beginning and continuing this journey with learners.

Challenges of Being a Preceptor

You are invited by your manager to be a preceptor. You are both honoured and terrified. If this is your first time formally in this role, then you have a lot to learn. To begin, recognize that becoming a really good preceptor takes experience, just as becoming a competent (even expert) care provider takes experience. Reading this chapter and other resources will help. You might be fortunate that the agency you work for provides preceptor education. The first step is to determine what is available in the form of lectures, workshops, preceptor manuals, et cetera and to engage with them before your preceptee arrives. You cannot possibly be fully prepared on the first day no matter how much homework you do, so begin with a positive attitude and a sense that you will learn every day through reflection, experience, and ongoing formal learning. Know that your apprehension is normal—with preparation, this apprehension can be lessened. With a positive approach, being a preceptor can be a fulfilling experience for you and a gift to a learner.

From the Field   *Learning Together*

I was delighted to be asked to be a preceptor! This would be my first time. I thought, "Wow, they think I am good enough to teach a new person—that's super!" My sense of excitement was soon drowned out by horror. What if I made a mistake? What if my student asked a question that I couldn't answer? What if . . . ? I didn't sleep a wink the night before our first shift together. I just did my best to have a positive attitude and kept reminding myself—my student and I will learn together.

BETH PERRY, PROFESSOR, FACULTY OF HEALTH DISCIPLINES, ATHABASCA UNIVERSITY

Once you overcome the initial challenge of self-doubt about your ability to be a preceptor, you can become aware of some of the realities and challenges faced by preceptors. One important challenge is that preceptors must balance the needs of preceptees with the needs of patients for whom they are caring and the realities of the workplace. Patients might be seriously ill (or become seriously ill during a shift), and work environments can have high staff turnover and other challenges (Hallin & Danielson, 2009). As a preceptor, you might feel torn between the needs of your patients and the needs of the preceptee. The reality is that patient safety always supersedes anything else. If you keep that in mind, then you will know what to do. If you do have to make a choice and the preceptee's needs are not addressed at that point, then explain the situation later to the learner and use it as a learning moment to help them understand priorities.

Not all students are going to succeed (at least not at first). You might have a learner who lacks appropriate knowledge, skills, and attitudes to perform safe, competent (for her or his level), and ethical care in the clinical environment. You might be the only line of defence for the patient, and your responsibility to, and advocacy for, the patient and society might become your priority. As Luhanga et al. (2008, p. 214) write, preceptors must be able to recognize and manage unsafe practices by students—preceptors are the "gatekeepers for the profession." If you have a learner who is disruptive and exhibits other problematic or unsafe behaviours, Luhanga et al. provide strategies gathered from preceptors with experience in such situations. Their first recommendation is to catch unsafe practices early or even prevent them if possible. A key first step is giving the learner a complete orientation to the learning environment and establishing clear expectations. Preceptors need to make their own expectations clear, ask learners about their expectations, and understand the expectations of the program before the learning experience begins. Clear expectations, understood by all involved, can prevent issues and problems. One preceptor in the Luhanga et al. study describes how she presents her expectations: "I try to nip it in the bud pretty quickly so as to prevent it. Upfront, I tell students what I expect. Like, I expect you to know every med you give. I expect if you don't know something to ask me, we'll look it up. I don't expect you to know everything, so don't feel pressured" (p. 216).

Actively involved preceptors often prevent problem behaviours and unsafe practices by learners by providing them with demonstrations, chances to practise, cues, prompts, and frequent feedback throughout the learning experience (Hendricson & Kleffner, 2002). Such active involvement of the preceptor, including close observation especially in the early days of the relationship, can give learners the best chance for success. As they gain confidence and competence, preceptors can step back and encourage more independence within agency guidelines. However, that initial investment of time and energy by the preceptor can be crucial as learners stretch toward practising at their full scope.

Preventing unsafe and disruptive behaviours is not always possible. If a learner is doing something that jeopardizes the safety of another person (or even himself or herself), then the preceptor must stop the behaviour immediately. Further actions (Luhanga et al., 2008) include (1) communicating concerns directly to the learner to determine whether the learner is aware of the problem, (2) working with the learner to set up a detailed plan for improving performance, and (3) involving the faculty adviser if the learner is a student.

Preparing preceptors for their role is important to the success of the preceptor-preceptee relationship. Ensuring that preceptors are enthusiastic about being preceptors is essential. Careful preparation can fuel this enthusiasm and prepare preceptors for positive outcomes from their preceptoring experiences, encouraging them to continue in this role. Hallin and Danielson (2009) note that, in some clinical environments in which students are preceptored, turnover is high. Preceptors might be placed in the role before they have appropriate orientation, appointed not because they are ready to be preceptors but because it is their turn. If you are asked to be a preceptor and do not, after careful reflection and self-assessment, feel safe in this role, then discuss your concerns with your manager before agreeing to it. Again, the principle of patient safety overrides all else.

Characteristics of Effective Preceptors

Research has been carried out on the qualities of effective preceptors in various health-care disciplines. Effective preceptors in pharmacy have professional expertise, actively engage learners, create a positive learning environment, are collegial, and discuss career-related topics and concerns (Huggett et al., 2008). Pharmacy students value preceptors whom they perceive as role models, who are interested in teaching, relate to learners as individuals, are available to provide direction and feedback, and spend time with learners (Young et al., 2014). Medical students note that effective preceptor behaviours include openness to questions, constructive feedback, enthusiasm, review of differential diagnoses, and delegation of patient responsibilities (Elnicki et al., 2003). Nursing learners value experienced, knowledgeable professionals who guide them to think critically and create a supportive and nurturing environment (Phillips, 2006).

Although these studies emphasize slightly different characteristics of effective preceptors, some commonalities are clear. First, excellent preceptors want to be preceptors or at least can be perceived as wanting this role. Students are attentive to the level of enthusiasm and support that preceptors bring to the relationship. Second, effective preceptors have expertise to share and do so willingly with learners. Learners appreciate preceptors who share their knowledge by involving them in the learning process: that is, preceptors who make learning interactive and two-way, challenging learners to think critically. Third, we can note openness, collegiality, support, respect, and nurturing. Students report learning best in a positive learning environment infused with these attitudes.

A Strategy to Try ▶ *How to Be Positive When You Don't Feel Very Positive*
This could also be called the "fake it until you make it" approach. You are human. You have days when you don't feel like being at work, let alone having a student with you. You have more than enough to do to get through the day, and you just don't have one ounce of energy left over to answer another question!

When this happens, forgive yourself. Remember that you do have limits. You can try to make an attitude adjustment—give yourself a little lecture and start fresh. If that fails, then just take one hour or even one moment at a time and try to be a positive preceptor. Fake your enthusiasm until, perhaps after one or two positive exchanges, your real enthusiasm might start to return.

Perry (2008) concludes that nurses who do their job well come to know that they are making a difference for patients (and in your case learners). This realization starts a positive cycle of feeling good about their work, trying even harder to do well, and feeling even better about their success in their role.

So, on those days that you just don't want to be a preceptor, fake it until you can get this positive cycle started. The result might be a great day after all!

What Helps to Make You a Better Preceptor?

You can use multiple strategies to become an outstanding preceptor. First, be sure that you have the support you need to succeed. Being a preceptor can be stressful, but you can be more effective if you receive support from faculty advisers, managers, colleagues, and clinical educators on the unit (Yonge et al., 2002). Support can come in many forms, including formal education programs and workshops through your agency, opportunities to meet with faculty advisers to learn about their expectations of a preceptor, discussions with colleagues about how they enhance their success as preceptors, or informal chats with clinical educators for teaching tips. You can identify the forms and sources of support most useful to your knowledge gaps. Do reflect on your needs and ask for the support that you need to perform your role well.

A second important strategy is preparation. Less experienced preceptors might feel unprepared for and unsure of their roles and responsibilities, adding to the stress of the role. Hallin and Danielson (2009) recommend that, in addition to the preparation outlined earlier in this chapter, preceptors confirm that they have clear guidelines on the expectations of their role and what students are allowed to do in clinical settings. They suggest that, in part to gain this knowledge and to learn the more subtle skills of being an effective preceptor, inexperienced preceptors be preceptored by experienced preceptors. This requires team preceptoring rather than initially being a preceptor on your own and can be effective for some individuals. In particular, new preceptors must be specifically prepared for student evaluation, which can be idiosyncratic to each student's agency, complex, and demanding.

A Strategy to Try ▶ *Consider Forming a Preceptor Support Group*
You can organize a group of preceptors in your agency for regular gatherings to share experiences, debrief problems, and engage in professional development on being an exemplary preceptor. You can meet in person or online through Skype or another real-time meeting software.

Set some guidelines for your group on the requirements for participation, frequency of meetings, nature of discussions, and so on. Just as in the learning environment that you are creating with students, so too the group should be a positive, supportive, nurturing, and engaging gathering. Confidentiality will be an important consideration. Give your group a catchy name, such as the Preceptor Partners or the Pre Ceptors, to instill a sense of togetherness and build group morale. Adding an element of food sharing or exercise (meet while you walk) can augment the group purpose.

THE PRECEPTOR-PRECEPTEE RELATIONSHIP

Being a preceptor is being a teacher. To succeed as a preceptor, you need to be skilled both as a clinician and as an educator. Previous chapters offer numerous clinical teaching strategies that you can apply as a preceptor. Following is a brief overview of some educational strategies that you might be able to incorporate into your role.

As a preceptor, developing an effective relationship with the learner is an essential starting point and critical to learning. The preceptor-preceptee relationship can be more effective with mutual respect and a demonstration that the preceptor cares for the learner as a unique individual. A warm welcome is the first step. The tone of the first interaction with the preceptee is important to the success of the relationship. A smile and pleasant tone set the stage for a mutually satisfying and respectful relationship and for optimum learning. If the initial contact is by telephone or email, then a pleasant welcoming tone is equally important. Something as simple as remembering (and using) the names of learners demonstrates respect.

Beyond a personal welcome, the preceptor must take steps to help the preceptee feel part of the team by introducing the learner to other team members (Hilli et al., 2014). An effective preceptor makes time for the learner to ask questions and become familiar with routines and the culture of the environment. Preceptees also need orientation to practical things such as the washroom location, what to do if they need to call in sick, break times, daily schedules, and idiosyncrasies of each workplace.

Trust is built over time. As a preceptor, your goal is to help the learner feel like a partner who evolves to function to the full extent of their skill and knowledge levels over time. Preceptors can build trust by seeing preceptees as valuable additions to the team, by being honest and saying "I don't know" if they are not sure of the answer to a question, and by being open to new ideas introduced by the preceptee (Vancouver Coastal Health, 2006).

Kramer (1974) described four stages of reality shock for new employee preceptees: honeymoon, shock, recovery, and resolution. These stages are a normal part of learning. In the honeymoon phase, preceptees are enthusiastic and full of energy that a good preceptor can encourage and harness. During the shock phase, preceptees might become unmotivated and discouraged and struggle with self-doubt. The recovery and eventual resolution phases see a cautious optimism resolving into a positive outlook. Excellent preceptors are mindful that learners can be at any of these stages during their time together. Being attentive to how learners are feeling and finding time to chat with them about what makes them anxious, excited, or worried can help to build a trusting relationship that poises the learner (and preceptor) for success.

A Strategy to Try ▶ *Create a Worry Quilt*

Sometimes people are reluctant or unable to share their worries with others, especially with a person in a position of perceived power such as a preceptor. Sensitive preceptors might notice a learner who expresses anxiety in clinical situations. You can chat privately with the learner to encourage the sharing of anxieties. One strategy that you could use prior to this chat is to have the learner create a worry quilt. You can ask the learner to create visual representations of things that are worrisome in the clinical situation. The learner places each worry on a quilt square and pieces them together into a quilt pattern. The quilt squares can be pieces of coloured paper, or they can be virtual boxes. What the learner puts into the squares can be words or images. When the quilt is pieced together, you and the learner have a visual depiction of the learner's major worries. Themes might become evident and lead to specific strategies for mitigating stressors. The constructed quilt can show that the learner is worrying about the same issue in different ways. Being able to address the worries expressed or condense them into one issue that can be addressed can help the learner to move forward. Below is an example of a worry quilt.

Things that worry me

IV starts	**making a medication error**	**hurting a patient**
getting yelled at by a doctor	**not knowing the dose of a medication**	

Figure 2. An example of a worry quilt

A Strengths-Based Approach

Preceptors can encounter difficulties in their relationships with students through personality or value differences or seemingly limited skill or interest of learners (Cederbaum & Klusaritz, 2009). A strengths-based approach focuses on learners' self-determination and validates the unique strengths that learners bring to their learning (Melrose, 2018). This can be a useful strategy for preceptors who encounter difficult relationships with learners (McCashen, 2005). In a strengths-based approach, the preceptor emphasizes discovering, enhancing, and promoting the interests, knowledge, and goals of the learner. The preceptor facilitates self-discovery and clinical reflection, creating a learning environment with mutuality and respect and a focus on strengths over deficits. If a strengths-based approach is used effectively, then learners feel empowered and affirmed. Some learners who are more familiar with a deficit model might feel uneasy at first if they expect a teacher-centred, top-down teaching approach. The strengths-based perspective can provide an innovative framework for working with students, one that emphasizes student empowerment, collaborative learning, and mutual growth (Cederbaum & Klusaritz, 2009).

How can preceptors enact a strengths-based approach? One strategy is to use a learning contract, as explained in Chapter 6. This contract can be verbal or written, outlining by mutual agreement the roles and responsibilities of the preceptor and preceptee and emphasizing the mutuality of the learning experience. Another strategy is to express concerns positively and frame the resolution of problems as adding to existing strengths rather than overcoming deficiencies. Preceptors who embrace strengths-based approaches view the clinical situation from the perspective of the learner and try to create a positive learning space (Cederbaum & Klusaritz, 2009).

A Strategy to Try ▶ *Catch Them Doing Something Right—and Tell Them*
Being a preceptor is a challenge. Getting caught up in a spiral of finding weaknesses and trying to think of creative ways to address them is unfortunately too easy. If you focus on the positive, then be sure to spend time and energy finding and praising the things that are done well. If you see something positive, then tell the person right away, and pause for a moment to relish the feeling of success.

Debriefing

Halfer (2007) calls debriefing a magnetic strategy for preceptoring learners. Preceptors can use debriefing as a teaching strategy and an example of guided discovery learning. Usually, debriefing is a short exchange between the preceptor and the preceptee after a caregiving experience. Ideally, debriefing occurs in a private and safe location away from others who are not involved in the experience (Wickers, 2010).

Debriefing has four elements: reflection, rules, reinforcement, and correction (Roberts et al., 2009). Initially, a preceptee is invited to reflect on their performance, giving the preceptor an opportunity to gain insight into the learner's perspective. This reflection requires learners to gather their thoughts and share them, often a learning experience in itself. Next the preceptor teaches general rules about the procedure, reinforces them, and corrects errant thinking expressed or demonstrated by the learner. Wickers (2010, p. 83) emphasizes that "structuring a seemingly unstructured learning event is paramount to the effectiveness of the debriefing session" and reminds us that positive support is part of the successful debriefing model.

Reflective Practice

Preceptors can use the instructional strategy of reflective time to enhance the consolidation of theory and practice (Duffy, 2009), encouraging students to assess their practice through guided reflection. Schon (1983) suggests that the capacity to reflect on action as part of engaging in a process of continuous learning is one of the defining characteristics of professional practice. Schon differentiates the capacity to reflect *in* action (while doing something) from the capacity to reflect *on* action (after you have done it). To elicit real reflection, the preceptor must ask appropriate questions that move the reflection beyond self-justification or self-indulgence. The desired result is learning or perhaps behavioural change or enhanced skills proficiency.

A Strategy to Try ▶ *Instant Replay Without a Camera*
Consider using a sports approach to encourage reflection on action. The instant replay allows athletes to review the effectiveness of their actions by watching videos of them. In a health-care interaction, the preceptor will not have a video camera in hand, but after the interaction the preceptor can invite the learner to replay (role-play) the scenario—creating an instant replay. By acting out the interactions, learners will have a chance to reflect on their actions. After the replay, the preceptor and learner can discuss what happened, lessons learned, and changes that the learner would make the next time.

THE EDUCATIONAL PROCESS: ASSESSMENT, PLANNING, IMPLEMENTATION, EVALUATION

The educational process parallels the health-care process with four stages or steps: assessment, planning, implementation, and evaluation. Preceptors need to spend time assessing the learning needs, goals, strengths, and limitations of each learner to be able to coach and guide the student to maximum learning. No two learners are the same, and thus skilful assessment helps to personalize the learning experiences that are facilitated by the preceptor. Although assessment is important at the outset of the relationship, it is also an ongoing activity for preceptors.

Excellent assessment sets the stage for planning instructional opportunities to meet the knowledge and skill gaps identified for each learner. After learning strategies are implemented, evaluation by the learner in consultation with the preceptor determines whether the knowledge and skill gaps have been addressed. If not, then further specific learning activities need to be sought to continue addressing learning needs and goals. Each evaluation feeds back into assessment, and the cycle continues.

The key to success in skilfully implementing this cycle is effective communication through building excellent rapport between the preceptor and the learner. Positive interpersonal relationships are the starting point for rich learning experiences in the clinical environment. A successful preceptorship requires honest and respectful interaction, particularly when the preceptor provides feedback or evaluation to the learner.

A Strategy to Try ▶ *Talk Out Loud*

One strategy for communicating clearly with preceptees is to talk to yourself. Talk out loud as you ask yourself how you are assessing patients, planning care, or implementing and evaluating the success of your intervention. Students benefit from hearing the preceptor's thought processes aloud (Smedley et al., 2010). No extra time is needed to complete a task if you include the verbal commentary yet hearing your thought processes provides learners with great learning—especially auditory learners.

THE REWARDS OF BEING A PRECEPTOR

Although being a preceptor is challenging, and partly because it is challenging, many professionals experience the role as stimulating. The most desired and frequent rewards are often non-tangible. The rewards that preceptors rank the highest are the ongoing learning that a preceptor achieves, opportunities to share students' enthusiasm for learning, and fostering professional skills, attitudes, and confidence in learners (Campbell & Hawkins, 2009).

In some cases, more tangible rewards are provided, depending on the agency involved. Campbell and Hawkins (2009) give examples of preceptors who receive continuing education vouchers; verification of hours toward recertification; a reduced price or free admission to museums, lectures, or cultural and sports events; certificates of appreciation; and opportunities to be part of research publications and presentations. Other institutions provide preceptors with paid time off or salary adjustments. As the competition for clinical placements and preceptors becomes more intense, considering some of these more tangible reward systems might be advantageous to clinical practice programs. If administrators and educators plan to offer tangible rewards for participation as preceptors, then preceptors must be consulted on what they consider appropriate and valued rewards. Most preceptors are motivated intrinsically and by altruism. They engage in this role because they have a strong desire to pass on their knowledge and skills to the next generation of caregivers.

A Strategy to Try ▶ *Ideas for Preceptor Rewards*

If you are an administrator or educator who seeks ideas for rewards that preceptors might find appealing, here are some creative ideas that you can consider (or ask preceptors what they would find rewarding):

- a plaque with a new inscription for each year that a person is a preceptor
- apprecigrams (handwritten notes of thanks)
- introduction of preceptors at convocation
- parking privileges
- adjunct professor status

CONCLUSION

Simply put, preceptors are vital. They are charged with the pivotal responsibility of helping learners to gain competence to deliver safe, autonomous, professional care. Preceptors have tremendous power to guide the development of professional practice and ultimately the success of learners in the health-care professions.

In this chapter, we offered an overview of the roles, challenges, and rewards of being a preceptor. We discussed several strategies to help preceptors excel. The foundation of all instruction as a preceptor is building a strong relationship with the learner. A caring relationship founded upon mutual respect and reciprocity is a prerequisite for a health-care learning environment. In such an environment, learners can thrive, and preceptors will be rewarded for devoting time and sharing knowledge, skills, and professional insights.

Health-care professionals have a responsibility as licensed team members to help others rise up to meet their potential (Eley, 2015). Preceptors have a responsibility to guide learners, to act as role models, and to lead others into the profession by preparing them to succeed (Hilli et al., 2014). Being an exemplary preceptor can be as rewarding for the teacher as it is for the learner. It is not a role that can be taken lightly. Preparation, reflection on and in action, and continuous learning are fundamental to becoming and excelling as a preceptor.

REFERENCES

Andrews, M., & Wallis, M. (1999). Mentorship in nursing: A literature review. *Journal of Advanced Nursing, 29*(1), 201–207.

Benner, p. (1984). *From novice to expert: Excellence and power in clinical nursing practice.* Jossey-Bass.

Boyd, R. D., & Myers, J. G. (1988). Transformative education. *International Journal of Lifelong Education, 7*(4), 261–284.

Brookfield, S. D. (2000). Transformative learning as ideology critique. In J. Mezirow & Associates (Eds.), *Learning as transformation: Critical perspectives on a theory in progress* (pp. 125–150). Jossey-Bass.

Campbell, S., & Hawkins, J. (2009). Preceptor rewards: How to say thank you for mentoring the next generation of nurse practitioners. *Journal of the American Academy of Nurse Practitioners, 19*(1), 24–29.

Cederbaum, J., & Klusaritz, H. A. (2009). Clinical instruction: Using the strengths-based approach with nursing students. *Journal of Nursing Education, 48*(8), 422–428. https://doi.org/10.3928/01484834-20090518-01

Dawson, p. (2014). Beyond a definition: Toward a framework for designing and specifying mentoring models. *Educational Researcher, 43*(3), 137–145. https://doi.org/10.3102/0013189X14528751

Dirkx, J. M., Mezirow, J., & Cranton, p. (2006). Musings and reflections on the meaning, context, and process of transformative learning: A dialogue between John M. Dirkx and Jack Mezirow. *Journal of Transformative Education, 4*(2), 123–139.

Duffy, A. (2009). Guiding students through reflective practice—The preceptors' experiences. A qualitative descriptive study. *Nurse Education in Practice, 9*(3), 166–175.

Eby, L. T., Rhodes, J., & Allen, T. D. (2007). Definition and evolution of mentoring. In T. D. Allen and L. T. Eby (Eds.), *Blackwell handbook of mentoring* (pp. 1–20). Blackwell.

Eley, S. (2015). The power of preceptorship. *RN-Journal.com*. https://rn-journal.com/journal-of-nursing/the-power-of-preceptorship

Elnicki, D. M., Kolarik, R., & Bardella, L. (2003). Third-year medical students' perceptions of effective teaching behaviors in a multidisciplinary ambulatory clerkship. *Academy Medicine, 78*(8), 815–819.

Gopee, N. (2011). *Mentoring and supervision in healthcare* (2nd ed.). Sage.

Halfer, D. (2007). A magnetic strategy for new graduate nurses. *Nursing Economics, 21*(1), 6–11.

Hallin, K., & Danielson, E. (2009). Being a personal preceptor for nursing students: Registered nurses' experiences before and after introduction of a preceptor model. *Journal of Advanced Nursing, 65*(1), 161–174. https://doi.org/10.1111/j.1365-2648.2008.04855.x

Hendricson, W. D., & Kleffner, J. H. (2002). Assessing and helping challenging students: Part one, why do some students have difficulty learning? *Journal of Dental Education, 66*(1), 43–61.

Hilli, Y., Salmu, M., & Jonsén, E. (2014). Perspectives on good preceptorship: A matter of ethics. *Nursing Ethics, 21*(5), 565–575. https://doi.org/10.1177/0969733013511361

Huggett, K. M., Warrier, R., & Malo, A. (2008). Early learner perceptions of the attributes of effective preceptors. *Advances in Health Sciences Education, 13*(5), 649–658.

Knowles, M. (1984). *The adult learner: A neglected species* (3rd ed.). Gulf.

Kramer, M. (1974). *Reality shock: Why nurses leave nursing.* Mosby.

Luhanga, F., Yonge, O., & Myrick, F. (2008). Strategies for preceptoring the unsafe student. *Journal for Nurses in Staff Development, 24*(5), 214–219.

McCashen, W. (2005). *The strengths approach.* St. Luke's Innovative Resources.

Melrose, S. (2018). Mentoring non-traditional students in clinical practicums: Building on strengths. *Journal of Clinical Nursing Studies, 6*(3), 39–45. http://www.sciedupress.com/journal/index.php/cns/article/view/12797/8108

Mentoring Resources. (n.d.). *Mentoring Resources* [Website]. Sponsored by the Institute for Clinical Research Education, University of Pittsburgh. http://www.icre.pitt.edu/mentoring/index.aspx

Mezirow, J. (1995). Transformation theory of adult learning. In M. R. Welton (Ed.), *Defense of the lifeworld* (pp. 39–70). State University of New York Press.

Myrick, F., & Yonge, O. (2005). *Nursing preceptorship: Connecting practice and education.* Lippincott Williams & Wilkins.

Perry, B. (2008). Shine on: Achieving career satisfaction as a registered nurse. *Journal of Continuing Education in Nursing, 39*(1), 17–25.

Phillips, J. M. (2006). Preparing preceptors through online education. *Journal for Nurses in Staff Development, 22*(3), 150–156.

Roberts, A. (1999). The origins of the term mentor. *History of Education Society Bulletin, 64,* 313–329.

Roberts, N. K., Williams, R. G., Kim, M. J., & Dunnington, G. L. (2009). The briefing, intraoperative teaching, bebriefing model for teaching in the operating room. *Journal of the American College of Surgeons, 208*(2), 299–303. https://doi.org/10.1016/j.jamcollsurg.2008.10.024

Sandlin, J. A., Wright, R. R., & Clark, C. (2013). Reexamining theories of adult learning and adult development through the lenses of public pedagogy. *Adult Education Quarterly, 63*(1), 3–23. https://doi.org/10.1177/0741713611415836

Schon, D. (1983). *The reflective practitioner: How professionals think in action.* Temple Smith.

Seneca the Younger. (n.d.). *Letters to Lucilius.* BrainyQuote.com. https://www.brainyquote.com/quotes/seneca_405315

Smedley, A., Morey, P., & Race, p. (2010). Enhancing the knowledge, attitudes, and skills of preceptors: An Australian perspective. *Journal of Continuing Education in Nursing, 41*(10), 451–461.

Smith, M. K. (2002). Malcolm Knowles, informal adult education, self-direction and andragogy. In *The encyclopedia of informal education.* www.infed.org/thinkers/et-knowl.htm

Vancouver Coastal Health. (2006). *Preceptor resource guide.* http://www.vhpharmsci.com/residency/resources/preceptor_resources_files/Preceptor%20Resource%20Guide-Supporting%20Clinical%20Learning.pdf

Wickers, M. p. (2010). Establishing the climate for a successful debriefing. *Clinical Simulation in Nursing, 6*(3), e83–e86. https://doi.org/10.1016/j.ecns.2009.06.003

Yonge, O., Krahn, H., Trojan, L., Reid, D., & Haase, M. (2002). Being a preceptor is stressful! *Journal for Nurses in Staff Development, 18*(1), 22–27.

Young, S., Vos, S. S., Cantrell, M., & Shaw, R. (2014). Factors associated with students' perception of preceptor excellence. *American Journal of Pharmaceutical Education, 78*(3), 1–6.